£12-99

Healthy Mother,
Better Breastfeeding

Other books by Francesca Naish and Janette Roberts

Healthy Parents, Better Babies
Healthy Lifestyle, Better Pregnancy
Healthy Body, Better Birthing

Also by Francesca Naish

The Lunar Cycle
Natural Fertility

Healthy Mother, Better Breastfeeding

Francesca Naish and Janette Roberts

Newleaf

Published in Ireland by
Newleaf
an imprint of
Gill & Macmillan Ltd
Hume Avenue, Park West, Dublin 12
with associated companies throughout the world
www.gillmacmillan.ie

0 7171 3281 1

Printed by ColourBooks Ltd, Dublin

First published in Australia and New Zealand in 2002 under
the title, *The Natural Way to Better Breastfeeding*,
by Doubleday, Australia, an imprint of Transworld
Publishers Division of Random House Australia.

A CIP catalogue record for this book is available from the British Library.

1 3 5 4 2

The information provided in this book is intended for general
information and guidance only, and should not be used as
a substitute for consulting a qualified health practitioner.
Neither the authors nor the publishers can accept any
responsibility for your health or any side-effects of
treatments described in this book.

It often happens that the universal belief of one age,
a belief from which no one was free or could be free
without an extraordinary effort of genius and courage,
becomes, to a subsequent age, so palpable an absurdity
that the only difficulty is to imagine how such an idea
would ever have appeared credible.

John Stuart Mill (1806–1873)

We dedicate this book to all those courageous women
who have always known that breast is best!

Contents

About the authors

About Janette

Jan was born in Sydney in 1947 and graduated from Sydney University with an Honours Degree in Pharmacy in 1968. Her career in pharmacy spanned almost twenty years but a growing interest in nutritional and environmental medicine led her to complete a postgraduate diploma in Clinical Nutrition in 1983. She retired from pharmacy before the birth of her first son in 1985, but by then she had developed a specific interest in preconception health care, which she has promoted on behalf of the British Foresight Association since 1987. Her first book, *Healthy Parents, Better Babies* (co-authored with Francesca Naish) was published in 1996. The sequels, *Healthy Lifestyle, Better Pregnancy* (1999) and *Healthy Body, Better Birthing* (2000) are in print throughout the English-speaking world and translations are scheduled in Spain and Belgium.

In 1998 Jan set up a Wellness Centre in Sydney which led, by a roundabout route, to her developing the Natural Parenting website for the www.chakra.net portal. Jan also designed the Chakra Baby programs that are offered at Spa Chakra in Sydney and Melbourne, and through her association with the Chakra Alliance oversees the provision of wellness services to individuals and corporations. She is a frequent guest on radio, TV and internet chat shows, yet still finds time to be a mostly stay-at-home mother for her two sons in the Sydney suburb of Balmain.

About Francesca

Francesca was born in England in 1946. She studied mathematics at Sussex University, but after arriving in Australia in her late twenties she established a Natural Birth Control practice in Paddington, Sydney. This grew into the Village Healing and Growth Centre, one of the first holistic health care practices in Australia. Since 1994 she has trained health professionals in the use of her unique Natural Fertility Management techniques, including 'Better Babies' preconception health care, and has recently established agencies in New Zealand, Malaysia, the United States and England. In 1995, after twenty years in clinical practice, she established the Jocelyn Centre in Woollahra, Sydney. This is the first clinic in Australia to specialise in natural methods for fertility management, reproductive health and preconception health care.

Francesca is a qualified naturopath, herbalist and hypnotherapist. She writes extensively for the press, appears regularly on radio and television and is sought after as a public speaker and lecturer. She also pioneered the teaching in Australia of natural vision improvement. She has written five previous books: *The Lunar Cycle* (1989), *Natural Fertility* (1991), *Healthy Parents, Better Babies* (1996), *Healthy Lifestyle, Better Pregnancy* (1999) and *Healthy Body, Better Birthing* (2000). The last three books were co-authored with Janette Roberts, and are now published throughout the English-speaking world, with translations being undertaken in Spain and Belgium. Francesca has two sons and lives in the Sydney suburb of Bronte with her family.

Acknowledgements

Francesca's thoughts

Once again, this book has most assuredly been a team effort. On behalf of us both I want to extend our deep gratitude to all at Random House and Doubleday, especially Katie Stackhouse, for their great support and enthusiasm, which keeps us on our toes. Our editor, Amanda O'Connell, brings as always her wonderful eye to our work and makes what we felt was good into something even better—thank you, Amanda, for your magic. Our illustrator, Deborah Clarke, once again enlivens these pages with her skill, and the yoga advice, as in our previous book, owes much to the expertise of Cheryl Dingle, herself a proud mother who attributes much of her success in childbearing and raising to yoga.

Liz Courtney, our agent, has continued to support us while breast-feeding her own two children. Thank you, Liz, and a big thank you to our wonderful cover girls, Isabella and (the other) Francesca, who manage to make all our books look so attractive.

My personal thanks go, as always, to my colleagues and staff at the Jocelyn Centre for Natural Fertility Management and Holistic Medicine.

Our team there is a constant source of inspiration, information and emotional and practical support. There is no way I could do what I do without them. Special thanks to Nicole Mason for the typing of my handwritten (and often illegible) first drafts. Nicole not only manages to read what I've written, but often what I intended to write too. Thanks also to Joan Coleman for tidying up my 'loose ends' and to Anna and Rod Brennan and their 'better baby' Oliver, who helped me write much of this book by supplying their mountain retreat for peace and quiet. To Malcolm Harrison, who kept things going on the domestic front and fed me, many thanks.

All of this would mean nothing if not for the work and support of my dear co-author, Jan. Once again, her words inspire me to produce my own best work and fill me with confidence that an audience will also be inspired to experience their own best breastfeeding. It's a great joy to work so closely with someone whose ideas, and their expression, are in such sympathy with what I feel and want to say.

However, I might have much less to say about breastfeeding if it were not for my own joyful and fulfilling experiences with my sons Albion and Sebastian, breastfed constantly and in all circumstances (sometimes to my mother's chagrin) for the first three years of their lives, and sporadically for yet another. It forged an unbreakable bond between us, was one of the happiest and most satisfying times of my life, and also the cause of much amusement. You'll read later on of how my first son entered his chauvinist piglet stage by pulling *Playboy* off the newsagent's shelf to the cries of 'Tit! Tit!'. The accompanying volume of *Wheels* (owing to his obsession with Matchbox toy cars) added to the public hilarity. Both my boys have grown to be loving, emotionally balanced and healthy adults who in turn bring joy to others, especially me.

Jan's thoughts

In all my earlier books I chose to acknowledge family, friends, professional colleagues, business associates, publicists and editors, not to mention a powerful past life connection, and, most importantly, my dear co-author.

This time, I still want to thank Francesca for all the usual stuff: a plethora of supporting research and journal articles which have at times led to frustration and a burning desire to do just that (burn the lot, that is), but that desire is always balanced by lots of laughter and her complete support—always. So thank you, dear Francesca.

However, this time it was really my two sons who played the major role in shaping the contents of this book. David and Michael, who breastfed for a grand total of ten years, who fed while sleeping and waking, while lying still and on the move, while happy and sad and certainly until they had had 'enough', taught me all I know about breast-feeding. I thank them both, and in their robust good health and emotional security and maturity I see the benefits every day in every aspect of all our lives. Together we did good, guys!

Note to readers

In this book we deal with both self-help and practitioner-guided treatments. If you are in any doubt about what you should do on your own or what requires professional help, always seek help. But be sure that the medical advice you receive is from a practitioner who has a commitment to using as natural and non-interventionist an approach as possible.

The herbs and supplements that we recommend will be available from a number of different sources including holistic and natural health practitioners, health food stores and pharmacies. Supermarkets also carry an increasing range of supplements and remedies, but wherever you purchase your products, make sure that they fulfil the dosages that we recommend.

In the case of nutritional supplements we have given clear guidelines regarding dosages for general use. Herbal and other natural remedies come in a variety of forms, and it is therefore not possible to give similarly clear-cut guidelines for dosage. Whether the product is a tablet, capsule, loose herb, fluid extract or powder, if it is sold through a retail outlet it will have clear directions for use on the container and you should follow those. If you are in any doubt or if you have specific concerns it is always advisable to consult a natural health practitioner. You can take a copy of our book to your practitioner for reference.

Throughout the text we have referred to your baby as 'he'. We would like to reassure you that our only reason for doing so is to distinguish easily between references to the mother ('she') and the baby. Though neither of us has been fortunate enough to have a daughter we would certainly have welcomed such an addition to our brood of delightful sons.

Finally, after 37 years of offering counselling and support to nursing mothers, and promoting breastfeeding throughout Australia, the Nursing Mothers Association of Australia (NMAA) has had a name change to the Australian Breastfeeding Association (ABA). All references to this important body throughout the text have been changed to their new name.

Prologue

Thoughts from Janette

In early 1999, David and Lindsey's first child was born. I met them initially when they attended Balmain Wellness Centre after reading about it in *Healthy Parents, Better Babies*. They were enthusiastic about the preconception health care message and were really diligent in following all of our recommendations. They gave copies of the book to all their friends who were planning to have a baby, and I even had a thank you phone call from one of their colleagues who was living in California at the time.

Lindsey followed the program all the way through her very healthy pregnancy, but within days of giving birth it appeared that all was not well. Her very alert baby didn't sleep for lengthy periods as she had expected he would. Finding it difficult to deal with his wakefulness and subsequent crying, she responded by wrapping him more securely and rocking his cradle constantly. She finally resorted to a dummy. These actions met with varying degrees of success (or failure, in Lindsey's eyes).

Eventually Lindsey and her very healthy, but not very sleepy, baby stayed for a week at a special facility for new mothers. There she was shown how to get him into a routine and how to get him to sleep using a method known as controlled crying. Her baby would soon tire of crying, the theory went. And the theory proved correct. After crying for the comfort that he needed, but which never materialised, he eventually stopped and fell asleep! But when I visited Lindsey I was distressed by her baby's cries and I could see that she felt exactly the same way.

At about the same time that this new mother was dealing with the early weeks of her baby's life in a way that was making it unnecessarily difficult for the whole family, another expectant mother gave birth. Tina had managed a very successful business before her baby was born. She ran a cafe and grocery store where everything she sold and all the food she prepared had one theme. The products were dedicated to achieving and maintaining good health: organic, chemical free and low in saturated fat and salt.

Three days after the birth Tina was back in the store, but her new daughter was nowhere to be seen. She told me that she was very lucky— she had a really 'good' baby, even though she hadn't been able to breastfeed her. But since she had tried hard, she certainly wasn't going to beat herself up about it. I couldn't help but wonder where she got the very odd idea that breastfeeding isn't something that everyone can do!

Lynette and Malcolm's first son was born after they had followed all the recommendations in *Healthy Lifestyle, Better Pregnancy*, yet by the time the baby was 8 months old, Lynette was ready to wean him. She told me that he suddenly seemed less interested in the breast, had bitten her on a few occasions, her menstrual cycle had returned and she was experiencing heavy bleeding and premenstrual symptoms. Her doctor had suggested that the only answer was a higher dose contraceptive pill, the low dose version of which she had been taking since just after the birth. She was overwhelmed by all of these complicating factors and very uneasy about the added hormones that her baby would receive if she chose to continue nursing. She felt that weaning was the easiest answer to her problems. I was sad that she did not consider that there might be alternatives to pharmaceutical methods of contraception for herself and to premature weaning for her son.

Another mother who had done all the right things before conception and during her pregnancy contacted me when her baby was just 10 weeks old. She was agonising over how soon she could start to give her daughter something more than breast milk, was uncertain about which foods were suitable as first solids and was also wondering how she should prepare them. She wanted me to write another book to tell her exactly what to do.

Four women with four fairly unremarkable stories. And during my twenty years as a community pharmacist and more than fifteen years promoting preconception health care and natural parenting many more have shared their doubts and concerns with me. These women's uncertainties have prompted me to ask myself the same questions over and over again.

- Why do so many women doubt their mothering abilities?
- Why are they reluctant to trust their intuition and their instincts?
- Why do they experience uncertainty when responding to their baby's fundamental needs?
- Why do they resist offering the easiest, most logical, most appropriate form of comfort?
- Why is it so difficult for women to follow a completely natural course through breastfeeding and beyond?
- Why are women unable to let their babies set the agenda through this period of rapid growth and development?
- Why so much uncertainty and lack of confidence at a time when a woman's maternal instinct should be most keenly honed?
- In short, why is mothering so difficult these days?

To find the answers to these questions and those that Francesca experienced in her practice, we decided to do what my friend had suggested. We knew that there should be another book in the *Better Babies* series. Like all the others, it deals with the natural approach to a perfectly natural function—breastfeeding. But it also looks at why many women experience difficulty, doubt and uncertainty about doing something that should come so naturally, and then looks at ways to make breastfeeding easy and uncomplicated.

Following your maternal instinct is important, so the book discusses ways to improve that instinctive response. When you follow those instincts, life becomes much easier for the whole family. When you respond instinctively, mothering becomes the simple, natural, joyful activity it was meant to be and you develop a stronger bond with your baby that translates into a more fulfilling relationship as he grows.

So if you're ever doubtful or uncertain about what to do, just remember that your child is undoubtedly your very best guide through his early years. Only he can really know what his needs are, and those needs are pretty simple—comfort, appropriate stimulation, food and drink. You can be certain that your child is very good at indicating what he needs and when he needs it and you can also be sure that your own physical, mental and emotional health is enhanced when you respond on cue to all those needs.

Thoughts from Francesca

Our principal motivation for writing this and our previous books has been to give expression to ideas and information that seem to us to be of undeniable importance. Daily, in my practice, I meet people who would (and do) benefit from the information in this, and our other, books. This motivates and inspires me to keep writing and reaching a wider audience. These same patients, and their needs, ensure that I'm constantly exploring new ideas and remedies—which end up in the books.

However, it seems to be a two-way experience, with unexpected rewards. Just as my experiences in practice contribute to the writing of the books, so their publication influences the way our clinic develops and the response of the women and men who attend it. As each book appears, it brings with it a greater level of acceptance, and my experiences in practice become more and more rewarding. I'm never quite sure whether I'm writing the books, or they are writing me.

When I first started out in practice over 25 years ago, my focus was on helping women and couples to use natural methods of contraception. Of course the same timing techniques (which you can read about in Chapter 9) that can be used to avoid conception can also be used to achieve it, and I soon became aware that there was a need for a 'conscious conception' program. This natural, holistic approach to fertility management, which includes natural medicine and remedies, provided the basis for my first book, *Natural Fertility*. The inevitable progression was into preconception health care and then into helping people overcome their fertility problems. The outcome of this was Jan's and my first joint book, *Healthy Parents, Better Babies*, a guide for preconception health care for both parents.

That has remained the focus of my practice ever since, but far too often I had the frustrating experience of seeing my patients improve their general and reproductive health, achieve a healthy conception and, having realised their immediate goal, revert to old habits and belief patterns. Frequently they would allow themselves to be persuaded of the need for intervention, not able to trust their own preferences for a natural approach to the management of their pregnancy.

Then Jan and I wrote *Healthy Lifestyle, Better Pregnancy* to ensure that the improvements that couples made in their health in order to achieve a healthy conception and their preference for a natural approach could continue to support both mother and baby through the next nine months. Once the book was published I found in my practice that more and more women and their partners followed through after conception with a natural approach during their pregnancy. It was as if the book gave them the confidence they needed to follow their preferred path.

The next challenge was to encourage women to continue to trust their instincts and opt for an intervention-free birth. So we wrote *Healthy Body, Better Birthing*, which gives women (and their partners) the support they need in order to make the choices that in their hearts they usually want to make.

Some of the promises of a preconception health care program are a much greater chance of a healthy pregnancy, trouble-free birth and successful breastfeeding experience, as well as an exceptionally healthy child. But all these outcomes depend on the good work that is put in before conception being carried on into pregnancy and beyond.

So with our latest book we want to make it truly possible for you to give your child the best possible start in life. My motives, of course, are partly selfish. I don't want the frustration of seeing all the good work that is done before conception and during the pregnancy, labour and birth compromised due to lack of information and support about the natural approach to a successful and lengthy breastfeeding experience.

Whether or not you've followed our natural approach from before conception, I hope you'll enjoy and benefit from this book. I hope that it will help to convince more and more new mothers (and fathers) that they can successfully breastfeed and that they can choose to use natural methods and trust their instincts, without depriving their children of the best care on offer.

My reward comes from the many healthy, glowing, well-adjusted children and their happy parents who visit our clinic, send us their stories and photos and are a living testimony to the efficacy of the approach we espouse, which is really no more than commonsense and traditional beliefs and practices, with just a touch of modern 'magic'. When I see the absence of chronic ill health, allergy, asthma and behavioural problems and hear about the infrequency of doctors' visits that characterises these 'better babies', I know that what we offer you in this and our previous books is not only valuable but vital if we are to protect the health of the next generation.

Thoughts from us both

First of all we want to reinforce the message of the normality of breastfeeding. If you truly believe that breastfeeding is a natural, uncomplicated process, you're off to a head start. Just a very short while ago (in evolutionary terms anyway) breastfeeding was a completely instinctive response to a child's needs for comfort, food and drink. It was also considered no more remarkable or noteworthy than digestion. Questions such as 'Should I breastfeed?', 'How do I breastfeed?', 'Is he getting enough milk?', 'Does she need to change sides yet?', 'When should I start to give him solids?' and 'Should she be sleeping through the night by now?' were as fatuous and unnecessary as any questions you might ask about the efficacy of digestive acids and enzymes and the progress of food through your gastrointestinal tract. Statements such as 'I tried hard but I simply had no milk' and 'It's not something that everyone can do—plenty of babies survive on formula' were equally unheard of. So you can breastfeed—just believe it.

Our book is also an affirmation that breastfeeding is really the only way to feed your baby. We're a little tired of the experts who trot out the old 'A woman mustn't be made to feel guilty if she can't breastfeed' dogma. Let's face it: in the past, if you didn't 'succeed' at breastfeeding, your baby was lucky to survive. Breast milk is the best source of food, drink and comfort, not just for your baby but for your older child too—believe that as well.

If this ease and simplicity in relation to breastfeeding seems improbable, we'd like to assure you that it's not. Nor is breastfeeding, in its elegance and simplicity, the end of the story. When breastfeeding is as uncomplicated, natural, warm and instinctive as nature intended, the relationship that you establish with your child is similarly natural, warm and instinctive. An uncomplicated, satisfying and extended period of breastfeeding is instrumental in establishing everything that comes afterwards.

So if you're looking for solutions to all sorts of problems, particularly obscure ones, you may not find the answers in this book. After all, we are not breastfeeding counsellors or lactation consultants and those authors are much more experienced in dealing with problems than we are. We're simply two health professionals with a rather passionate interest in matters reproductive and a very strong commitment to the natural approach to these matters. We're also two mothers with many years of first-hand experience breastfeeding our own children, so we have mentioned a few problems that do crop up with monotonous regularity and we've also mentioned natural ways of dealing with them.

We won't graphically detail the anatomical features of your breast, the baby's mouth and tongue in relation to your nipple or the correct 'latch'. We'll talk about correct positioning because it's very important, but we'll also tell you that a healthy baby, left to make his own way to the breast after a completely natural, unmedicated birth will attach himself correctly. Our earlier book *Healthy Body, Better Birthing* tells you the best way to ensure that you and your baby get that sort of birth.

We'll emphasise that going with your instincts means trusting that your baby has reasonable needs rather than 'selfish' wants and that he also has his own unique timetable. If nothing else, this is the major theme of this penultimate volume in our series of *Better Babies* books. So rather than an endorsement of routines, timed feeds, scheduled feeds, dropped feeds and substituted feeds, we'll suggest that you let your baby indicate the frequency and duration of feeding.

We won't give you a fixed date for starting solids. Instead we'll tell you that your baby will indicate when it's time for something more than breast milk. When he does we've got lots of ideas about what is appropriate finger food for him. We're not going to tell you when you should wean him either because infant-led weaning will be different for each individual child.

We won't talk about ways to get your baby to sleep through the night. When you follow your baby's lead you'll almost certainly find that the whole family sleeps together and that your baby will continue to nurse through the night for some considerable time. That constant night-time contact should extend to constant physical contact during daylight hours as well, which simply means carrying your baby close at all times.

We recognise that we face different challenges today from the ones that our forebears faced. In our increasingly technological world we are subjected to alarming levels of toxins and pollutants which affect our growing children through their food and environment. So we've also made recommendations in the book on how you might protect the health of your breast milk and your baby from these modern problems.

So in telling you what we will and won't do you can see that our book is quite different from a lot of others. We have lots of positive ideas that will allow you to perform the most natural, most womanly, most important function without hesitation, without question and without doubt. We simply suggest ways of mothering and nurturing that have stood the test of time, but which have fallen from favour with our amorous embrace of science and technology.

Maternal instinct matters

We might surprise you by beginning our book with a discussion of maternal instinct, rather than with a description of the mechanics of breastfeeding (although we'll get to that shortly). But we firmly believe that a better breastfeeding relationship, and better mothering and nurturing in all the years that follow, begin by applying a very healthy dose of maternal instinct. There are other things you can do too to make breastfeeding a positive, enriching experience, and we'll talk about all of them in due course, but when you're able to follow those instinctive responses you're off to a flying start. Unfortunately, maternal instinct is often the last thing that today's new mother brings to breastfeeding (and to the early years) to both her own and her baby's detriment, not to mention the detriment of her family and the community.

What exactly is this much touted maternal instinct? Why is it often in short supply? In what ways is its absence detrimental? How can it be rekindled? What are the benefits of acting on instinctive responses? These are questions that we'll endeavour to answer in this book, and by doing so we hope to give you the best possible chance of experiencing rewarding and fulfilling years with your growing baby as well as an exceptionally happy, healthy, and emotionally well-adjusted child.

WHAT IS MATERNAL INSTINCT?

How many times have you said to yourself, 'I just *knew* I shouldn't have . . .'? At some time in your life, and certainly at some time during your years as a parent, you will know without any doubt that you have made an unwise decision. The reason you can say, 'I just knew . . .' with such conviction is your certain knowledge that you ignored an insistent inner voice when you made your original choice. That inner voice is your instinct. It is a powerful urging that guides you constantly, yet usually you are completely unaware of it (at least when it's operating properly). In the past, acting instinctively kept you alive (out of reach of the sabre-toothed tiger) and ensured the survival and wellbeing of your children, but you now rely less and less on your instinct to stay away from harm.

Unfortunately, in this age of information and technological overload, those instinctive responses that should kick in big time when you become a mother may be absent, or if they're present you may not trust them. You may even ignore them. So if you're wondering where your maternal instinct has gone, don't worry, you're not alone. If you're having great difficulty tuning into those responses, relax, it's just one of the challenges of being a parent today.

> Julia   My 35 years (13 as a flight attendant) were lousy preparation for mother-hood. I hadn't even changed a nappy, let alone prepared three meals a day, and I also had totally unrealistic expectations about how new babies behaved. My maternal instincts have really taken some awakening, but 7 months down the track I'm pleased to say I'm finally getting there.

WHERE DOES MATERNAL INSTINCT COME FROM?

There was a time when mothering came to all women naturally and instinctively. This happened when communities were much smaller than they are today, when everyone belonged to an extended family and had close and constant contact with all the members of that family. Then you would have been absolutely familiar with the whole continuum of pregnancy, birth, breastfeeding, weaning and nurturing, having supported your female kith and kin through it all. By the time your first baby arrived, mothering would have been second nature to you. The method of nurturing was uniform throughout a community, although it may have varied from culture to culture.

Conception and pregnancy were considered absolutely normal, natural, unremarkable events. For countless years, births occurred at home and were the exclusive domain of the women of the community who supported the labouring woman both physically and emotionally. No one doubted that a woman left to labour at her own pace was perfectly capable of bringing her baby into the world with very little outside help. After the birth, when placed on his mother's belly, and using the same pushing reflex that propelled him from the womb, the newborn would find his way to her nipple, attach and begin to suckle. This suckling stimulated the release of hormones that caused the uterus to contract and bonding to take place. This process was perfect in its design and elegant in its simplicity.

The new mother and her baby were then cared for and cosseted, spending several weeks in seclusion from the general community. This was considered an important time for the new mother to regain her strength and for her to get to know her infant. In traditional societies, the baby was carried close and constantly during his early months. In some cultures, his feet were not allowed to touch the ground for his first two years. This constant and close contact fostered an exquisitely intimate relationship that allowed a mother to respond to her baby's signals immediately and appropriately. Sensing when he was about to urinate or defecate, she would simply hold him away from her body to avoid soiling. Existing as part of a dyad (rather than as one of two separate individuals), a woman answered her baby's needs with as little forethought as she answered her own.

Carried close during daylight hours and nestled beside his mother in the family bed, the baby would suckle and sleep completely at will. Nursing for short or long bursts and sleeping for short or long spells throughout the day and night, never separated from his mother, the baby rarely cried. A breastfeeding baby was an absolutely normal sight. Even today, cultures that forbid women to show their faces allow them to expose their breasts to nurse their babies, a fact that seems distinctly perverse to Westerners!

The comfort and nourishment the baby received at the breast were free of time constraints and when he was given his first taste of solid food it was almost incidental, since breast milk continued to be his prime source of nutrition until well into his second year (perhaps even later). Then his mother would probably have chewed the food first to make sure that her salivary enzymes had done some of the work of digestion. Her child would probably continue to nurse until well into his fourth or fifth year, when he would wean himself.

> Nicola   I just wish I'd never heard about 'controlled crying'. Letting my baby cry himself to sleep was the most distressing thing I've ever had to do. I knew it couldn't possibly be right because it made me feel so terrible. It took me a while to stop worrying about what everyone would say, but when I finally took Jack into bed with me, I was so much happier and he was so much more settled, I just knew we'd got it right.

Questions were never asked about a woman's ability to breastfeed, let alone to feed for an extended period—it was simply something that the vast majority of women did, and did without thinking or questioning. Infant survival (and a very effective method of child spacing as well) depended on feeding a baby in this way. Of course there were cases of lactation failure (after a famine for example) and also of women wanting to be free of the physical restraints of nursing (so there is nothing new under the sun). In such cases the service of a wet nurse was enlisted, and if that was unavailable, the baby might have been given raw milk from a grazing animal or a similarly poor substitute of some sort of ground grain mixed with water. While wet-nursing was a legitimate and effective substitute for milk from the biological mother, the same could not be said for the various artificial substitutes, and frequently the baby would not survive these offerings. Since agricultural and pastoral communities are a relatively recent phenomenon, only developing about 10 000 years ago, it should be apparent that breastfeeding has been the primary method of nurturing a baby for most of humankind's time on this planet. Of the world's 4237 species of mammals, homo sapiens is the only one threatening nature's method of caring for its newborns!

But back to the story . . . Children spent their early years surrounded by close family members, never separated from the ebb and flow of family life. Lactating mothers often nursed each other's babies and took turns at caring for toddlers while keeping an ever observant eye on older children's activities. These activities were unstructured and usually involved play with household items or very simple wooden toys. Young children were quickly enlisted to help with household chores and to look after even younger children. Everyone, from the youngest sibling to the most senior grandmother, mothered a child in much the same way. That way, which was how things had always been done, was simply an instinctive response to the growing child's needs rather than a response to some authority's preconceived ideas of what a child should need or do.

WHERE DID MATERNAL INSTINCT GO?

Loss of the extended family

For hundreds of thousands of years, this elegant and simple story repeated itself in countless communities around the globe. Now, however, the extended family has largely disappeared from Western civilisation, although it is still alive and well (but probably under serious threat) in many less developed countries. In today's society, births are usually attended by specialist health professionals (and quite often the woman's partner), but are much less frequently witnessed by female family or friends (although we're pleased to say that's changing).

Many women have never seen their mother, aunts, sisters, cousins or friends nurse a baby. Those role models who are available often prefer to nurse discreetly behind closed doors, particularly if it's a very mobile toddler who's helping himself to a breast. With the huge increase in women in the permanent workforce, few spend any significant time caring for young children. Consequently, the modern woman who has an intimate knowledge of birth, breastfeeding and babies before she has a child of her own is the rare exception rather than the rule. It's hardly surprising that breastfeeding is no longer the natural, uncomplicated activity that it once was and that modern women no longer respond intuitively or instinctively when they become mothers.

Information overload

An over-abundance of information on every conceivable aspect of parenting must also take some of the blame for the absence of instinctive responses (meae culpae). Today, you are surrounded on all sides by a plethora of authorities offering advice that may not only be contradictory, but may also be in direct conflict with what your inner voice is telling you. No wonder you doubt the wisdom of that voice (if you can even hear it). And as if the volume of information already available was not enough, it has grown exponentially with the advent of the information superhighway.

To top it all off, more information, in the form of advice (often unsolicited) comes from mothers, mothers-in-law, friends and family members who, more often than not, are themselves prior recipients of inappropriate advice. This is in direct contrast to the traditional wisdom and tried and true practices that older mothers could once impart or demonstrate to younger women.

> **Angela**   For weeks I tried the advice of everyone who proffered it. First it was the hospital staff, then of course my mother and mother-in-law had plenty to offer. It never occurred to me to do *exactly* what I felt like doing every time Eliza cried. When I finally gave up rocking, wrapping, and patting, removed the dummy and simply nursed my daughter, we never looked back.

But you continue to read, look, listen and ask questions, because you've been conditioned to believe that logic and reason (not to mention trendy psychological theory) should prevail and that a thoughtful, considered, left-brain answer is the correct one. Meanwhile, the instinctive response that comes from the right side of your brain struggles to be heard. It's an insistent nagging voice that, when ignored, gives you an uncomfortable feeling in your gut, yet more and more it wages a losing battle with your analytical, thinking side. Dr Caroline Myss, a wise and erudite woman and author of *Anatomy of the Spirit*, summed up the problem: 'Your mind is a bullshit artist, only your heart tells the truth.'

The consumer society

Once, just about the only thing that you needed after the birth of your new baby was some cloth to bind him close to your body. Now, the separation that began at a baby's birth is encouraged and assisted by the purchase of a multitude of baby accessories. Most couples approach the birth of their child only after having prepared a separate nursery, equipped with all manner of specially designed furniture and other accoutrements in a range of vibrant colours and designer materials and fabrics. This is seductive stuff and rampant consumerism at its worst. Prams, strollers, bassinettes, change tables, cots, highchairs, swings, bouncinettes and playpens are just some of the 'prerequisites'. Bottles, teats, dummies and sterilising equipment add to the list, but most of these items are unnecessary and only serve to reinforce the separation that makes it very difficult to tune in to your maternal instinct and to accurately intuit your baby's needs.

Nutritional factors affect maternal instinct

Finally, at a much more fundamental level, there are specific nutritional factors that have a profound bearing on the presence (or absence) of instinctive response. An adequate supply of the trace elements zinc and manganese is necessary for maternal instinct, and a deficit has been shown to cause animals to neglect their young. Maternal instinct also works best if your baby enjoys robust good health. But increasing numbers of children suffer from subtle problems that can make instinc tive mothering very difficult indeed. For example, a zinc deficient baby who cries excessively and is difficult to settle will be unlikely to evoke an appropriate maternal response in his zinc deficient mother, who is probably suffering from postnatal depression. Unfortunately, due to present farming practices and a number of common lifestyle factors (including the prior use of oral contraceptives), your body may be short of both zinc and manganese. We'll look at ways of rectifying deficiencies in Chapter 5.

HOW CAN MATERNAL INSTINCT BE REKINDLED?

So if you're finding it hard to tune into those instinctive responses, there are good reasons. But there are several things that you can do to reconnect to your maternal instinct, and not surprisingly they're also important for a successful and long-term breastfeeding relationship, not to mention your continuing good health and that of your baby during his early years.

- Sometimes it's useful to ask yourself, 'What would a woman from a traditional society do?' While we can't go back to tribal ways, we can learn a lot about our baby's needs by observing older customs and practices. Always remember, that your baby only has 'needs', not 'wants'.

- If the procedure you're offered or the advice you're given makes you feel uneasy, stop for a moment. Ask yourself, 'What is my gut feeling?' Silence the left, thinking part of your brain and listen to your inner voice.

- Put yourself mentally into each situation. Try to focus on how you really feel with each decision. One choice will probably give you an uncomfortable feeling of doubt and concern and the other an inner feeling of rightness.

- Often you will find that your first, perhaps subliminal, response is the right one. It's just a question of banishing the doubt that can set in as you strive to do the best for your baby. Try to stick with that first response, before it is overwhelmed by your need to respond in the way the 'experts' advise.

- Focus on your love for your child. The reason instinctive response is such an integral part of mothering or parenting is that it is triggered by your deep need to protect your offspring. This sets the situation apart from most other modern experiences and the intensity of your feeling for your baby is the most effective way to initiate your instinctive response.

Run through these simple exercises whenever you're confronted with a choice and the more frequently you do this, the more attuned you become to those instinctive responses that have guided women for millennia. Take the time to develop and nurture your maternal instinct— it's much wiser than you think—and when you heed that inner voice, mothering becomes a much easier and more joyful experience.

SCIENCE AND SOCIETY THREATEN BREASTFEEDING

Now bring your instinct to bear on this question. Imagine that the world had invented a new dream product to feed and immunise everyone born on earth. Imagine also that it was available everywhere, required no storage or delivery, helped mothers to plan their families and reduced their risk of cancer. Then imagine that the world refused to use it! At the end of a century of unprecedented discovery and invention, even as scientists discover the origin of life itself, this scenario is not, alas, a fiction. The dream product is human breast milk. (UNICEF: *Take the baby-friendly initiative*)

Quite simply, but quite certainly, breastfeeding is now an endangered practice around the world. In the West, the majority of women are breastfeeding on discharge from hospital, but the number of women still nursing their child on his first birthday barely exceeds 10 per cent. Ironically, the nearer a mother is to a modern hospital, the greater the pressure to stop breastfeeding! Breastfeeding rates are also in decline in the less developed nations and the average length of the breastfeeding period is a fraction of what it once was. Not surprisingly, the reasons for this decline are very closely tied to the reasons women have lost touch with their maternal instinct.

The scientific approach

The technological revolution saw a concurrent rise in the belief that everything in nature could be improved upon and many theories were put forward on how this improvement could best be achieved. Dr Truby King was one example of these theorists, and even though he advocated breastfeeding right from the start (rather than the much favoured honey mixed with breadcrumbs!), he also advocated scheduled feeds and solitary sleeping. These ideas are, unfortunately, still with us today, more than 200 years later.

At about the time that technology started the climb towards its ascendancy, men also became involved in the birth process. Our earlier book, *Healthy Body, Better Birthing*, discusses this history. Having planted their feet very firmly in the doorway leading to traditional women's business, it wasn't long before men were offering their two cents worth on the conduct of all related issues. All would have been well if what they advocated had been seen as a mere two cents' worth. But they brought emotion into the equation, saying that women who chose to ignore their 'scientific wisdom' were risking the physical and emotional health of their children. Nothing much has changed, since the same old argument is trotted out today if a woman questions the need for intervention during pregnancy, labour and birth, not to mention breastfeeding, and nothing is better designed to strike doubt into the heart of a mother than an implied threat to her baby.

So women were told by the 'experts' (usually male) that babies were selfish creatures who benefited from a regular schedule, timed feeds and not too much attention, since it could lead to spoiling. Sleeping together was a dangerous custom as a mother could 'overlay' her baby, and damage or even kill him.

These so-called 'experts' brought about profound changes in breastfeeding practices in a very short space of time. These changes included the introduction of breast milk substitutes based on cow's milk (which was, thanks to industrialisation, being produced in excess and in need of a market) as well as the rigid regimens and timetables for feeding and sleeping that bore no relation whatsoever to a baby's real needs.

Along with these profound changes in traditional practices came graphs, charts, normal distribution curves and a plethora of other useless information. This was supposed to be solid scientific evidence documenting the behaviour, weight gain, sleeping and waking times and much more of babies who were in completely abnormal situations, fed on a diet which was never designed for them. Some of this irrelevant information still appears in modern medical, nursing and midwifery texts and consequently is advocated by some doctors and other health professionals.

Fortunately, we're slowly regaining an understanding of nature's infinitely wise design, and we are also more cognisant of the problems that arise when we tamper with nature, but this is still far from being a universal trend. The 'expert' voices have not diminished in volume nor have they been short of ever more innovative, trendier theories, although theories have regularly risen and fallen from favour throughout the years. Aphorisms such as 'A baby must cry, he needs to exercise his lungs' and 'If he's crying he simply needs to be wrapped more tightly' are thankfully now out of vogue, but 'controlled crying' is with us still.

The potential to consult 'experts' and to use medical technology at every stage of your reproductive life from conception onward inevitably affects your ability to respond instinctively to a situation and to breast-feed successfully. You may no longer trust your body to conceive, bear, give birth to and nourish a child, believing that IVF is an acceptable way to conceive, and that routine ultrasound, CVS and amniocentesis are prerequisites for a pregnancy that proceeds normally. You may also be convinced that high-tech monitoring and medical intervention alone can ensure the birth of a live, healthy baby, and believe that infant formula, administered to a set schedule, is an acceptable substitute for the nour-ishment and comfort that your baby receives at the breast. Because you've been told that science and modern technology can provide all the answers, you can easily be convinced that the technological approach is the way to go. And if your instinct isn't blinded by science, it still has to face a possibly even tougher foe—the expectations and pressures of modern society. Let's look first at how these factors combined to promote the acceptance of formula feeding.

The rise of formula feeding

When forceps and chloroform were introduced to the birthing scene, it was initially only the wealthy classes that could afford to avail them-selves of these scientific marvels. In the same way, pure, white flour (devoid of nutrients but aesthetically more pleasing than the coarse, brown, unrefined product) was something to which only the aristocracy had access. The lower classes aspired to those things that the upper classes could afford, since their acquisition indicated an upward move in the social hierarchy. So it was with formula feeding—since the upper classes could afford this scientific marvel, they embraced it, and since the lower classes could not, they wanted it. Furthermore, what the upper classes were avidly embracing must surely be superior as they must know a thing or two, mustn't they?

Jan saw this at first hand when she worked, during the 1980s, as a pharmacist in Sydney's Chinatown. The new Asian immigrants took to formula feeding with a vengeance, seeing it as a progressive step, indicative of their 'Westernisation'. Breastfeeding was considered an activity reserved for the peasants and lower classes.

Tragically for the one and a half million babies who die every year due to the use of infant formula, and for the countless others whose health is compromised, the belief that a bottle is better than the breast has not been limited to upwardly mobile Westerners.

The multinational corporations that discovered a ready market for the excess cow's milk that the world produces have not only had a hand in the decline of breastfeeding, but can be said to have had an extraordinarily damaging effect on the health of children in the Third World. Advertising slogans like 'The Way a Doctor Cares and the Way a Mother Loves is the Way Mead Johnson Feeds' are extraordinarily emotive, but devoid of any sense of ethics or morality. This same dissimulation serves to protect such advertising campaigns from laws that are put in place to prevent bottle-feeding being portrayed as superior to breastfeeding. When 78 per cent of the human population lives in conditions that Westerners would not tolerate (e.g. no access to running water), breastfeeding provides a measure of protection from the gastrointestinal conditions that can kill. Ironically these may well be caused by using contaminated water and inadequately sterilised equipment to make up formula. But advertising is simply the handmaiden of the technology and corporate greed that has been responsible in a more subtle way in the West for the decline of breastfeeding and the maternal instinctive response.

Social and cultural expectations

Even though many of the practices that the so-called experts once advocated and that women followed slavishly for so long have been shown to have detrimental effects on both mothers and babies, many of them, such as timed and scheduled feeding and separate sleeping quarters, are still around in one form or another since they have become very much the social and cultural norm. Consequently it's often quite difficult to challenge or to overturn what is considered socially and culturally acceptable. It takes a fair amount of courage and strong conviction to feed and nurture your baby in ways that are in direct opposition to the ways chosen by most of those around you.

Cultural expectations of women have changed dramatically too. Not so very long ago, when a woman married she was expected to devote herself to home and family. These days, it's more a question of how many weeks (did anyone suggest months?) before she can return to the coal face. It's not politically correct to become simply a stay-at-home mother. Rather, just as soon as she can, a woman is expected to take up the career that she left off before she had her baby. The idea that the new infant might need more constant attention from his mother is very threatening in contemporary society, where individuals of both sexes are redefining their roles and expectations.

Current social attitudes are divided, as are the expectations, desires and needs of many new mothers. When a mother puts her child into care out of necessity, she can suffer feelings of guilt or inadequacy. When she puts her child into care out of choice, in order to pursue other personal goals, she may be accused of neglect.

While we certainly don't wish either of these states upon you, we do feel strongly that all choices, especially those that have a bearing on something as important as your child's wellbeing, should be made in an informed climate, and with the understanding that your child cannot negotiate his own needs. Then, given your available options, you need to make the best choice for both of you. If you are feeling guilty, that won't help your baby, so you need to achieve the right balance.

Part-time work and more flexible working hours are acceptable answers to the dilemma of many women who wish to spend time with their babies, but also need to earn income, further their careers and engage in stimulating adult interaction. Although the number of women in part-time work continues to grow by demand, very little has been done by government or employers to formalise these arrangements and protect part-time employees from the loss of entitlements. Fathers who choose the option of part-time work meet with even less sympathy. For any couple trying to fulfil both their parental and work roles with some degree of satisfaction, sacrifices will inevitably need to be made. We can only hope that the importance of your relationship with your baby is given its rightful place at the top of the list when you make your decisions, ahead of the new car or the overseas holiday.

With the demand for equal opportunity for women and the economic need many mothers have to contribute to the family's finances, childcare centres have proliferated and are now regarded as a necessary adjunct to women achieving equality. They are also the only available support for many mothers who work. In Australia, over half of all women who have children below four years of age are in the labour force. This is not surprising, given that a family in 1995 needed to earn 1.6 times the income of a similar family in 1970 to maintain the same living standards. With the number of working mothers constantly increasing, and with the loss of the extended family, significant numbers of children are in care for a great portion of their early lives. It has been calculated that a child can spend up to 12 500 hours in care before beginning formal education.

It's clear that some childcare centres are better than others, and you need to choose carefully if you require their services, but however good the care is, fewer hours in contact with your baby inevitably affects the supply of breast milk and your chances of breastfeeding success. It also affects the degree of intimacy that you have with your child and this can significantly compromise your intuitive maternal response.

ENHANCING THE MATERNAL INSTINCT

Your maternal instinct has the best possible chance of being heard when you give birth to an optimally healthy baby in just the way that nature intended and when breastfeeding is quickly and easily established. It's further enhanced when the bonding period is undisturbed and when your baby feeds as often and for as long as he wants. (See our earlier books for more on how to achieve a better pregnancy, birth and bonding). Both the breastfeeding relationship and those instinctive responses are most likely to succeed when the whole family sleeps together and when that night-time contact is extended to include constant physical contact during daylight hours as well. So it's not really very difficult, but it's certainly a little different from the advice you might receive from other sources. But if you believe that past gener-ations of women had wisdom to impart, then you're ready to hone your instinctive response. Of course that response will tell you that breast milk is best, but let's back that up now with some facts and figures!

Breast
is best

'Breast is best' is much more than just a catchy phrase. It is a statement which, in its simplicity, accurately sums up the act of breastfeeding. Breastfeeding is best for your baby, for you, and even for society in general. We'll be looking at why we can assert this so confidently throughout this chapter.

BEST FOR YOUR BABY

Breast milk is species specific

The reason why breast milk is unquestionably the perfect food for the young of the human species is that it is designed specifically for them! All milks contain hundreds of different factors that are present in varying proportions depending on the type of mammal from which the milk comes. This extremely variable composition means that each type of milk is perfectly adapted for the growth and development of the young of that particular species. Cow's milk is the perfect food for calves, goat's milk the perfect food for kids (but not of the human variety), camel's milk is the perfect food for baby camels and human milk is the perfect food for human babies. There's one notable exception to this rule: soya milk is not the perfect food for baby soya beans (and is not the perfect replacement for human milk either—more of this in Chapter 8). Not surprisingly, the milk of the great apes—chimpanzees, gorillas and orang-utans—most closely resembles human milk.

While all mammalian milks contain four basic constituents—protein, fat, carbohydrate (sugar) and water—it's the varying proportions of each of these components that distinguish one from the other.

Breast milk contains digestible protein

Milks from fast-growing species contain a high proportion of protein, unlike the milk of slow-growing species such as humans. For example, rat's milk contains twelve times more protein than human milk, and cow's milk four times more.

The primary protein in cow's milk is casein and levels are 300 times higher than in human milk. Casein forms tough, rubbery curds that are hard for your baby to digest and the high protein concentration is a big load for his immature kidneys to handle. On the other hand, lactalbumin, the whey protein in breast milk, forms soft, easily digested curds that your baby can readily metabolise. The reason a breastfed baby's nappies have no unpleasant odour is that the protein in human milk is completely broken down to the last amino acid, leaving no residue to cause offence.

Two particular amino acids that are found in breast milk are worth mentioning. Cystine enhances overall growth and taurine is particularly important in the development of the brain. Both are vital for your baby's optimal physical and mental development, yet have only recently made their way into infant formulae.

Breast milk is low in fat

The fat content of various mammalian milks differs as well. Human milk contains relatively little fat compared to milk from other species that are dependent on their fat stores for survival. The milk of elephant seals, for example, has a higher fat content than butter, simply because the baby elephant seal is nourished by its mother's milk for four weeks only. In that short space of time, the baby must grow from its birth weight of about 35 kilos to its weaned weight of close to 135 kilos. Amazingly, during those four weeks, the mother seal eats nothing at all, so for all intents and purposes she simply converts a huge slice of her own blubber into the blubber that covers her baby.

The type and content of fatty acids found in milks differ too. The long chain polyunsaturated fatty acids that are typical of human milk have a number of very important functions, including the production of highly active biological substances that are vital for the normal working of your baby's body. They also form the major part of the cell walls of every single cell in that body and are essential for his brain and eye development. Studies have shown conclusively that breastfed babies are smarter (by about 8 IQ points) than those that are bottle-fed, probably due to the presence of DHA (docosahexaenoic acid). DHA is one of the most abundant lipids in the brain and lipids account for 70 per cent of grey matter.

Formula manufacturers are now debating the necessity (or the wisdom) of including these fatty acids in their artificial products. Hardly surprisingly, the concentration found in the milk of an Inuit mother whose diet contains a preponderance of fat, is quite different from the concentration found in a mother from the African desert regions. So how much fatty acid to add (and exactly which ones) remains a conundrum. In the meantime, breastfeeding mothers know that their milk will contain the right amount of the right types.

Another benefit of the particular composition of fats in breast milk is that your baby is unlikely to become obese, either as a baby, a child or an adult. This reduces the risk in later life of cardiovascular disease, diabetes and other health conditions that are linked to obesity.

Breast milk has sugar for brain power

Human breast milk tastes exceptionally sweet. So don't blame your husband's passion for Maltesers and Mars Bars for your child's sweet tooth! (Actually, studies show that breastfed babies have fewer sugar cravings as young children and, therefore, fewer dental problems than bottle-fed babies.) This 'sugar of milk' found in such high concentration in human milk is lactose. It's a combination of two simple sugars— glucose and galactose—and delivers twice as much energy as glucose to your baby. Additionally, there are about 130 other sugars in human milk, making it very different from the milk of most mammals (not to mention formulae).

One of these sugars, known as NANA, is important for brain development. The brain also needs fuel for all its functions and this is supplied exclusively by glucose. Your baby's brain development is rapid in the last trimester of pregnancy, and continues at a great rate for the first three years of his life. That brain has unique needs. Although it only provides 10 per cent of your baby's total body weight, it uses 60 per cent of the energy he takes in through his food. Since the human brain is the largest of all the mammalian brains, it's not surprising that your breast milk is the sweetest milk of all. The provision of an abundant and constant source of fuel for the brain means that breastfed babies are more alert and more easily aroused than bottle-fed babies. This means your baby may be wakeful and may not fit the stereotype of the 'good' baby who sleeps for hours, feeds briefly and sleeps again. But console yourself with the fact that your wakeful, breastfed baby will also probably walk earlier and be better co-ordinated than a bottle-fed child, and his long-term brain development will be superior.

The high sugar (and low protein) content of human milk also means that a breastfeed won't sustain your baby for very long. A baby fed on a cow's milk substitute can go a lot longer between feeds. If you remember that the unique composition of human milk means that your baby will want to feed frequently, you're off to a head start in following your intuition when it comes to nursing 'schedules'.

Lactose, the sugar of milk, is an interesting molecule and confers some special properties on breast milk. Lactose and calcium are bound in such a way in human milk that every molecule of calcium is absorbed (unlike the much less efficient absorption from cow's milk, despite its much higher calcium content). Lactose does the same for the trace elements copper and zinc. Lactose intolerance is unusual in babies (as we'll explain in Chapter 8) so don't be concerned that this could be a problem.

Other nutritional advantages of breast milk

Zinc, iron and iodine are essential for brain development, and breast milk provides them in the most easily assimilated form.

Nature also makes sure that nothing in breast milk is wasted. Iron is garnered and incorporated into a compound called lactoferrin, ensuring that your baby absorbs every molecule of iron. In her in-genuity, nature has devised a dual function for this molecule. In lacto-ferrin the iron is bound, making it inaccessible to the iron-dependent, pathogenic bacteria that are the cause of gastrointestinal upsets. By contrast, artificial formulae contain no readily absorbable forms of iron (or any other nutrient for that matter).

This ready availability of iron in milk substitutes is one of the factors that places bottle-fed children so much more at risk of gastrointestinal disease. Together with the absence of the immune potentiating factors found in breast milk and a lack of potable water in developing countries, it contributes to artificial formula's responsibility for the death of 1.5 million children every year.

No need for extra water with breast milk

Human milk has a very high water content. This, combined with the low protein load and a sodium content that is significantly lower than cow's milk, means that fully breastfed babies don't need to be given additional water. Even in the hottest weather, if your baby is allowed to feed just as often as he wants to, he will remain adequately hydrated. Of course you should increase your intake of purified water, especially on very hot days, and avoid soft drinks, alcohol, coffee and tea (more on that in Chapter 6), all of which have a diuretic effect, increasing your output of urine and leading to compromised hydration levels.

Breast milk boosts immunity

Breast milk contains a variety of immune potentiating factors. Colostrum, the yellow fluid that is secreted in the days immediately following the birth, is particularly rich in immunoglobulins. One of these, secretory IgA, protects your baby by coating his gut wall and by promoting his immune system to produce its own IgA. The level of IgA remains high throughout the whole period of breastfeeding and is approximately ten times the level found in cow's milk or formulae.

Mature breast milk contains numerous other factors that boost your baby's immune system. These include B cells, T-cells, neutrophils and macrophages. Other protective factors, such as antibodies and gamma interferon are also present, and lysozome, an anti-infective enzyme, is found in concentrations up to 5000 times greater than those found in cow's milk. Those 130 sugars we spoke of earlier are important too: they substitute for the sugars on the cell walls where pathogenic organisms usually attach. All of these factors ensure that your breastfed infant is protected from a host of diseases and infections, such as ear and eye infections (that can lead to deafness and blindness) and gastrointestinal and urinary tract infections, until his own immune system has matured. They also put him less at risk of developing asthma, eczema, allergies and intolerances. He is also less likely to develop conditions such as coeliac disease later in life.

It is a sad fact that formula-fed babies are seventeen times more likely to suffer from gastrointestinal conditions than breastfed infants and fourteen times more likely to die from them. The increased rate of illness in bottle-fed infants is the same in Western countries as it is in the third world, the only saving grace being the improved level of medical care to which those children have access. Bottle-feeding increases the rates of diabetes, leukaemia and SIDS. It is also the cause of one million cases of otitis-related deafness annually in China, responsible for 60 per cent of infant deaths in Brazilian shanty towns and the cause of increased birth rates amongst those women whose only method of contraception is lactational amenorrhoea.

Breast milk is easy to digest

We've already talked about the easily digestible protein found in breast milk, but digestion is further aided by the presence of enzymes that make the nutrients more easily available to your baby. Another aid to digestion comes to your baby from your nipples. Towards the end of your pregnancy, bifidus bacteria (one of the many types of lactobacilli that live in a healthy gut) start to grow on your nipples. (Don't be alarmed, it's not an unsightly growth.) As your baby suckles and swallows, these good bacteria colonise his gastrointestinal tract, aiding his digestion and setting the scene for a lifetime of healthy gut activity. The lactobacilli provide further protection against gastroenteritis, diarrhoea, constipation and colic.

Hormones, growth factors and more

Breast milk contains a host of other compounds including growth factors and hormones. One of these, gonadotrophin releasing hormone, is present at ten times the concentration found in the mother's bloodstream. In the human adult, this hormone acts on the gonads and has a role in adult sexual behaviour, but we don't really understand the role it plays in the newborn. We assume that it and other polypeptides have a role in signalling to the immature brain and organs of your baby how they are to continue to differentiate and develop.

And it seems that breastfeeding results in better health throughout the individual's lifetime. Breastfed babies develop less atherosclerosis than bottle-fed infants, and the longer breastfeeding continues, the lower the adult cholesterol levels. Breastfed babies are also less likely to develop diabetes or multiple sclerosis.

Breast milk changes to suit baby's needs

Colostrum

Not satisfied with all these goodies and advantages, nature designed breast milk to be a living, changing fluid. Colostrum, which is secreted during the early days after the birth, has properties that are ideally suited to your newborn baby's unique needs. The laxative effect of colostrum rids the baby's gut of meconium, a mixture of mostly bile and mucus that is expelled shortly after birth (the baby's first bowel movement), and the bifidus factor then promotes the growth of friendly bacteria. Colostrum contains high concentrations of beta-carotene (this is responsible for colostrum's bright yellow colour), vitamin E and trace minerals. Cholesterol is also found in high amounts in colostrum. This molecule has a role in the development of brain tissue and its presence in the early breast milk may contribute to more efficient cholesterol metabolism in adult life. The protein content of colostrum is three times higher than that of mature milk, providing adequate nourishment during your baby's early days when he grows extremely rapidly.

Transitional milk

When the production of colostrum ceases, the transitional milk comes in and is produced from about day 7 to day 14. Transitional milk has reduced levels of immunoglobulins and protein and increased levels of lactose and fat, making it richer in kilojoules. Levels of water-soluble vitamins are increased and levels of fat-soluble vitamins are decreased.

Mature milk

After about day 14, mature milk comes in and will continue to be produced just as long as the baby continues to suckle. The law of supply and demand regulates the production of milk: the more frequently and strongly your baby suckles and the more milk he gets, the more milk you produce (and vice versa of course). In the early months of breast-feeding, despite widely differing maternal diets and levels of nutrient intake, the quality of women's breast milk remains within reasonably narrow limits. Breast milk is the most energy-dense food available; your baby would have to eat extremely large quantities of solid foods to get the same nutrition that he receives at your breast.

But after those early months, if you're not well nourished, your nutritional reserves can become depleted. Then the drain on your dwindling resources may compromise the quality and the quantity of the milk. So if you're planning a prolonged breastfeeding relationship (and we certainly hope you will be by the time you've finished reading this book), it's vitally important that you follow our dietary guidelines in Chapter 5.

It's also recognised that women on typical Western diets—low in quality protein and high in simple carbohydrates—produce milk that is particularly high in lactose. Although lactose is an important constitutent of breast milk (as we discussed earlier), too much of it can cause babies to suffer from colic, so this is another very good reason to follow our dietary guidelines.

Breast milk changes during the feed

The composition of breast milk also changes during a single feed. Your baby receives high concentrations of lactose in the foremilk to satisfy his immediate pangs of hunger or thirst. As he continues to feed and to drain the breast, he gets the hindmilk which is high in protein and fat. This helps to make him sleepy. The varying composition of milk during a feed is the reason that we recommend you follow the one feed, one breast rule. If you alternate the breasts during a feed, your baby may miss out on the rich hindmilk and the excess levels of lactose in the foremilk may make him unsettled. This may be an impossible (and unnecessary) rule to follow as your baby matures and can help himself to your breast, but we'll talk more about that in Chapter 3.

Breast milk changes to suit 'premie' babies

Even more remarkable is the fact that the composition of breast milk varies, depending on whether your baby is born at full term or not. The nitrogen content of breast milk is 20 per cent higher if you give birth prematurely, and the increased protein better meets the needs of a vulnerable 'premie' baby. The milk you produce if your baby is born early also contains more growth hormone as your baby obviously has more growing to do.

Breast milk provides more than nutrition

The words breastfeeding and breast milk denote nutritional nourishment, so it's easy to forget that your child receives a great deal more than food and drink at your breast. Recent studies have confirmed that the experiences to which your child's brain is exposed in the first three years, when it is still being formed, influence how it operates for the rest of his life. Just as it's vital that the correct nutrients for brain development are present (as in your milk), so it is critical that your child is given the kind of supportive emotional experience that breastfeeding can offer.

Breast milk provides comfort

Your baby receives comfort every time that he nurses. Sucking stimulates pleasure receptors in his mouth, so it's not surprising that a great deal of his sucking is unrelated to hunger or thirst, but simply done because it makes him feel good. Also, if you always nurse your baby according to *his* schedule, not some predetermined timetable, he receives positive reinforcement of his value as a person and enhanced feelings of security and belonging every time that he comes to your breast. Birth-educator and author Janet Balaskas writes: 'The feelings of satisfaction and pleasure at the breast are so blissful that constant repetition of these experiences imprints itself indelibly on a child's personality.'

The close contact involved in breastfeeding also allows your baby to continue to hear your heartbeat, which provides him with a continuum of experience from inside the womb.

Touch is important

Your skin is the largest sensory organ as well as the most primitive. Your baby's sense of touch is the earliest sense to develop. The earlier a function develops, the more important and fundamental it appears to be. So you could spend your life deaf and blind and lacking the senses of taste and smell, but you could not survive at all without the functions performed by your skin. Touch is something that every human being needs in order to become an emotionally healthy individual. Studies made over a century ago of orphan children who were never touched showed that the children did not thrive and sometimes even failed to survive. This tells us that your baby has an exquisitely sensitive need to be touched.

Nature takes care of this need while your baby's growing in the womb. There he receives constant stimulation of all his touch receptors. The level of stimulation increases with uterine contractions becoming stronger as labour progresses and reaches a peak as your baby makes his journey down the birth canal. This stimulation is vitally important because it appears to prime your baby's systems for their existence outside the womb and also seems to affect the satisfactory development of many of his senses.

The need for tactile stimulation doesn't finish with the birth. However, if things are allowed to unfold as nature intended, all will be well. By simply breastfeeding your baby you ensure that all the touch receptors on his body are constantly stimulated. So if it's possible, particularly in the early days after the birth, it's best if you and your baby are both naked while you breastfeed.

While it's obviously not always possible to continue in this natural mode once you're back to your normal routine, you should try to ensure maximum skin-to-skin contact as often as you can. This means avoiding nursing bras with a trapdoor through which your baby can suckle. Not only are these exceedingly unattractive garments, but they restrict the access to your naked flesh that is so important to your baby.

Breastfeeding improves co-ordination

As your baby grows you'll notice that he not only likes to stroke your naked skin but will also play with your exposed nipple. This constant fiddling and twirling is like some sort of infant five-finger exercise and has positive implications for the development of your baby's fine motor co-ordination.

The breastfed baby also receives both physical and visual stimulation from alternating sides as he shifts from one breast to the other. It seems that this is important for the neurological development that allows him to determine left from right. If your baby is bottle-fed it's unlikely that you'll shift him from side to side since your left or right-handedness will ensure that you cradle him on your most comfortable side. Sadly, a baby old enough to manage his bottle by himself may sometimes be propped in his pram or cot and left to feed himself, which means he'll get little stimulation of any sort.

Breastfeeding for sound facial development

Breastfeeding ensures the correct development of facial and dental structures (you've probably noticed the wonderfully full, chubby cheeks of breastfed children), and breastfed children are much less likely to suffer from speech difficulties than bottle-fed infants.

Breastfeeding fosters independence

During your child's early years he learns to cope with an extraordinarily complex world. He masters a multitude of skills and learns to develop self-control and good manners. But, because he is immature and inexperienced and because his control and understanding of his world is incomplete, even a happy, well-adjusted child will experience a great deal of frustration and tears. It's very easy to restore an unhappy, frustrated child to calm and good humour by breastfeeding him. The sucking makes him feel good, and what's more it seems that breast milk contains a sedative-like substance, possibly designed for just this purpose. The substance has been discovered in the milk, though not in the blood, of mothers who were not themselves taking any type of sedative. This suggests that the substance may be manufactured in the breast itself.

Breastfeeding is the easiest and most natural way to attend to any of the hurts, upsets, disappointments or fears that may be part of your child's early years. Events like a separation, a serious illness or a death in the family can be very stressful for a young child. He may be too young to fully comprehend what is occurring, he may not be articulate enough to tell you how he is feeling, but you'll certainly sense his distress. The comfort and security that you can offer him at your breast at times like these can be invaluable.

Breastfeeding is the best and easiest way to ease your child's transition from babyhood to security and independence and this reason alone should be sufficient for you to continue to nurse him beyond infancy. As he matures and gains some mastery over his environment (as well as over himself), as he learns to share, to be patient and to co-operate, he will no longer need to nurse. But in the years before this happens, he will be best served by a continuing breastfeeding relationship.

Benefits beyond childhood

All the hiccups that accompany the various milestones in your child's early years can be soothed more readily if you've both had the benefit of breastfeeding. Studies indicate that breastfed babies tend to be more content as they mature, and suffer less from fear, jealousy and spite than those who are bottle-fed. But a good relationship with teenagers, during those notoriously difficult years, isn't just happenstance. Feelings of mutual trust and respect, which are vital for communication during the teen years, have their foundations in the trust and respect that is initially established during a successful, fulfilling and long-term breastfeeding relationship.

BEST FOR MOTHERS TOO

The mothering hormone

It's not just your child who will benefit or be soothed by the act of breast-feeding. Prolactin, the hormone responsible for lactation, has some pretty amazing qualities—one of them is the ability to calm a hassled mother at the same time that she is calming her distraught child. Prolactin is known as the mothering hormone. It has also been called nature's Valium. When prolactin is coursing through your veins you'll be patient, more caring and generally more in tune with your baby than you might otherwise be. Nature seems to have made special provision for those years when, attending to your baby's constant needs, you become a candidate for sainthood. See Chapters 4 and 9 for more on the rela-tionship between prolactin and stress.

Happier baby, happier mother

Of course if your child is calm, you will also be more relaxed (and then your milk will flow more easily). Studies show that breastfed babies cry less and feel more secure, and this adds up to a much better experience for you too. Bonding is enhanced through the close contact, both physical and emotional, that is easier to achieve if you breastfeed, and a well-bonded, secure and happy baby means an easier and happier time for the whole family.

The benefits to your baby's health and intelligence that we've described will also improve your quality of life, and that's not to mention how his improved digestion and absorption will lead to less smelly stools, making nappy changing a relatively pleasant experience.

Pleasure for you

Special receptors in your baby's mouth make breastfeeding a pleasurable experience for him, but nature didn't forget about you! The hormone oxytocin, responsible for the let-down reflex, is the same hormone that is released at orgasm. So breastfeeding your baby makes you feel pretty good too. And what's more, in the same way that it helps you respond to your lover, oxytocin ensures that you constantly touch, caress and cuddle your baby. It probably doesn't need emphasising that nature's plan for mothers and babies is perfectly designed to ensure that everybody gets exactly what they need!

What about fathers?

Maybe nature gave modern fathers a slightly less than perfect deal, because sometimes her solution doesn't sit very well with today's social and cultural mores. Think about it . . . you're having a hit of oxytocin a dozen times a day or more, especially in the early weeks. While some lucky women say they achieve orgasm while breastfeeding, most women certainly don't (though Jan's and Francesca's friends must have wondered during their combined 18 years of breastfeeding their children). However a lot of women would definitely admit to feeling little need for sexual encounters while they're nursing, particularly when their baby is very young. Again nature has stepped in to ensure that the newborn gets exactly what he needs. This simply means no chance of a sibling until the first baby has received adequate nursing and nurturing.

On the other hand, some women feel especially sensual while they're feeding and their heightened sense of wellbeing (and perhaps a lack of anxiety about pregnancy) makes them very responsive to their partners as well as to their babies. We'll talk more about the complex interaction between sexuality, fertility and relationships in Chapter 9, but would like to mention here how this benefits you, as well as your newborn, by delaying your next conception.

Nature's contraceptive

Your baby isn't the only beneficiary if you can defer the arrival of your next child. You've probably got enough on your plate right now and could also do with a break before your next conception. You certainly need time to replenish the nutritional stores that pregnancy and breast-feeding have depleted, ensuring that your next pregnancy and birth will be as healthy as possible. In this way, your next child also benefits, as his health depends on your (and your partner's) nutritional status before conception and in the following months, and years, as you act as his larder.

Luckily, nature has all this in mind, and though breastfeeding is not an infallible method of contraception, it has a valuable role to play. In fact it's the most widely practised form of birth control throughout the world. The World Health Organisation estimates that each year unre-stricted breastfeeding prevents more unwanted pregnancies than all other contraceptives combined, and for 120 million mothers across the world, breastfeeding is the only available contraceptive. In Chapter 9 we'll also look further at the issue of contraception during breast-feeding—how it can be achieved and the role of prolactin and other factors in postponing the return of fertility—but unrestricted breast-feeding is critical to this process. It seems to be particularly important to feed your baby ad lib throughout the night if you want to prevent ovulation recurring.

Since breast milk remains the major source of nutrition for your baby as he grows into a toddler, the system that nature has devised helps to ensure that you only conceive another child once your first becomes relatively independent. As your child receives more and more of his nutrition from solid food and becomes sufficiently emotionally secure to nurse less frequently, your menstrual cycle is more likely to return.

A return to your pre-pregnant state

The delay in the return of your menstrual cycle also means that you have a chance to rebuild your iron stores. Even if you maintained these during pregnancy the demand on them has been high, and your baby's need for iron increases as his own stores start to become depleted. The last thing you need while nursing a new baby is iron deficiency and the fatigue that it generates.

The early involution of the uterus and a return to pre-pregnancy weight are two further benefits commonly attributed to breastfeeding. Due to the production of oxytocin during breastfeeding, your uterus returns quickly to its pre-pregnant state, thus reducing the risk of post-partum haemorrhage. In most breastfeeding women, the extra demand on kilojoules means that you regain your figure more quickly than if you bottle-feed.

However, Jan's experience led her to a slightly different conclusion about the return to pre-pregnancy weight. She was at her leanest (and slightly less than her pre-pregnant weight) within days of giving birth to her sons. In both cases, within 4 weeks of giving birth, she had acquired a ravenous appetite and some 7 to 8 kilos. She did not shed that extra weight until many years later when her younger son finally weaned. When he did, the weight fell off as quickly as it had appeared.

Jan's theory is that nature likes nursing mothers to have a bit in reserve in case the crops fail. Of course nature hasn't yet learned that the chances of mothers in developed countries experiencing a lean year are extremely remote. While Jan's theory is untested, we include it for those breastfeeding women who struggle to get their weight down. However, we don't want to give you an excuse for an over-weight state. If you've read our earlier books you'll know that we believe many women gain an excessive amount of weight during pregnancy. If you follow our dietary recommendations, your weight gain (and subsequent loss) will be just right for you and will stabilise to provide the right amount of fat reserves to sustain both you and your breastfeeding baby.

Breastfeeding protects against disease

Breastfeeding protects you against osteoporosis and ovarian and pre-menopausal breast cancer. It seems that the longer you breastfeed, the more protection you receive.

Breastfeeding is convenient and practical

Finally, at the risk of sounding flippant, we add that breast milk won't go off over the weekend, it requires absolutely no preparation and comes at the perfect temperature (which is a Godsend in the middle of the night), the cat can't get at it and it comes in pretty cute containers! In fact, it's convenient, sterile and cheap, all of which adds up to a whole lot of practical advantages for you.

In fact, breast milk is not only cheap, it's free! Formula, bottles, teats and sterilising equipment all cost money, and they also consume time. Not only do you have the hassle of buying, cleaning and sterilising equipment, but whenever you leave your home you have to pack it all up, transport it, unpack it, get it home, and find somewhere to store it. You'll certainly need an extra kitchen cupboard in which to house it.

With breast milk you'll certainly avoid the following scenario at three o'clock in the morning. You realise you haven't prepared enough formula, you try to wake your partner to take over, fail miserably, shuffle off to the kitchen, startle the dog (who wakes any other children who have finally decided to sleep through the night), you spill the milk, mop it up (or decide not to) and finally traipse back to your baby who, by this time, has become apoplectic. Alternatively, you might decide to pick your baby up and take him to the kitchen with you, in which case . . . we won't bother to list the potential disasters awaiting a sleepy mother trying to prepare formula with a screaming baby in her arms. How much easier to roll over, draw your baby (who's sleeping with you) to your breast and let him drink his fill as you drift gently through semi-wakefulness in the comfort and warmth of your bed.

Another practical advantage, and another major intellectual challenge you won't have to face, is trying to work out how much milk your baby will need. He will determine this himself. Because of nature's wonderful system of supply and demand, the more he needs, the more he suckles and the more you produce. What could be easier? The supply is simply regulated by the length and duration of the feeds.

Breastfeeding brings fulfilment

The most important advantage of breastfeeding for you, the mother, is the fulfilment that you will feel as you experience skin-to-skin contact with your baby, and the satisfaction of knowing that you are supplying life-giving food for him, just as you did all through your pregnancy via the placenta. Breastfeeding can and should be an automatic and easy continuation of this process of nurturing that began in the womb, and the knowledge that you can provide this, as nature intended, is your greatest reward.

SUBSTITUTES CAN'T COMPETE WITH BREAST MILK

Why, if breast milk is all these things (and every year scientists reveal further benefits), would women seek a substitute? And make no mistake about it, alternatives to breast milk have been around for a very long time. Some anthropologists believe that the domestication of animals such as cattle, goats and sheep occurred primarily to provide the means of feeding infants. The infant may have suckled directly from the animal's teat or been given the milk through a horn or from a skin container. One such container, fashioned in the shape of a breast, has been found in the ruins of a culture that dates back 3500 years. Interestingly, despite the fictional Tarzan, there are no records of humans being suckled by one of the great apes.

Sadly, a mummified infant lying next to a similarly preserved breast-shaped container in a Shanghai museum leaves us in little doubt that lots of infants who were fed breast milk substitutes died. They were either unable to digest the cow's or the goat's milk, or they may have caught a disease directly from the animal. Other breast milk substitutes such as water mixed with grain to form a sort of gruel were even less likely than raw animal milk to nurture and sustain a baby. In other words, until fairly recent times, the artificial feeding of infants was a disaster.

Undoubtedly, the most successful substitute for mother's milk is the milk of another mother. In the past, wet-nursing was considered an honourable profession and the children of royalty were often considered kin to the biological children of the mother at whose breast they nursed. These days, of course, wet-nursing has disappeared from Western society, a victim of our mania for hygiene and our phobia about cross-infection.

Of course modern day formulae are a far cry from the raw milk of grazing animals or the breast of a surrogate mother, but they obviously fill a need that has been with womankind for centuries. Many women want freedom from the demands of a constantly nursing infant. Other women feel that they produce insufficient milk to satisfy a ravenously hungry baby (or babies). Some women have a partner who resents the infant's demands on *his* breasts. Yet other women discover that breast-feeding is not a completely sensual and pleasurable experience. Those women whose nutrition is not adequate may have nipples which crack and bleed. All these types of women have been around for a very long time, so if you find yourself in any of these situations, you may also find some comfort in the fact that other women have been through it all before.

But if you're reading this book, then you're obviously looking for more than comfort in the failure of women of earlier generations to breastfeed. And by and large those failures were a very small fraction of the total. For the most part, women fed freely, unselfconsciously and completely successfully, a fact borne out by the burgeoning human population!

Despite many new developments and innovations in artificial formulae and the reassuring statements made by their manufacturers, none of these products can hope to imitate nature. Not only is breast best for your baby, it is best for you, best for the whole family, best for the community and best for the planet. The resources required to graze cattle, which involves the destruction of forests, to transport milk, which involves petrol consumption and the pollution of traffic exhaust, to manufacture formula feeds and the equipment they require such as bottles and teats, which involves the use of energy and the production of waste, and finally the disposal of these artifacts, which involves the pollution of large tracts of land are enormous and they are also unnecessary.

Breast milk is an extraordinarily complex substance, and the interactions and psychological development that accompany the act of breastfeeding are equally complex. Quite simply, it is presumptuous of us to think that we could manufacture a substance that could duplicate breast milk and that a bottle could replace the interplay and exchange that occurs when a baby nurses at his mother's breast.

So there are many compelling reasons why you should breastfeed your child, but equally important should be the recognition that breast milk is not just good for babies. However, many women experience enormous difficulty in establishing and maintaining breastfeeding. In Australia, more than 85 per cent of women are feeding on discharge from hospital, but only 10 per cent continue to do so beyond their child's first birthday. Yet, worldwide, the average length of the breastfeeding period is 4.2 years.

The reasons for lactation failure and early weaning in Western society are numerous. They include poor nutrition, an unhealthy lifestyle, ignorance, misinformation, health professionals who lack commitment to breastfeeding, cultural and social norms and changing work patterns. So let's look now at what you need to do to succeed at breastfeeding, because your 'success' will give your baby the best chance of achieving optimal physical, mental and emotional development. Let's look at how you can make breastfeeding easy—just the way it's meant to be.

Making breastfeeding easy

Now you know exactly why breastfeeding is best for you and your baby. Later we'll look at what to eat, how to exercise and all the things you need to avoid to ensure that breast milk passes stringent quality control. But there are some other things you need to know first. So in this chapter we'll look at the basics: how to breastfeed and how to make a positive contribution to a better breastfeeding experience.

WHAT'S HAPPENING TO MY BREASTS?

Often, one of the first signs of pregnancy is an increase in the size of your breasts. You'll also find that they become very tender, due in part to their increased blood supply. As your pregnancy advances, the areola and nipple tissue will darken in colour. It's thought that this darkening gives your baby a very obvious target area for attachment and also ensures that he takes the whole areola into his mouth rather than just the nipple.

The small protuberances (Montgomery's tubercles) that surround your nipple are oil-producing glands and they also increase in size and become more active. The sebum that they secrete during pregnancy and lactation lubricates and protects your nipples. This protective effect is enhanced, from quite early in your pregnancy, by the production of colostrum. This is the first breast milk. It's bright yellow in colour, full of antibodies and perfectly suited to your newborn baby's growth requirements. The transitional milk, which follows colostrum, lasts until about day 14 when your mature milk comes in.

The hormones that maintain your pregnancy also prepare your breasts for nursing. Hormones continue to play a role after the birth, with prolactin responsible for milk production, and oxytocin (produced during labour and at orgasm) responsible for the let-down reflex. You'll experience this as a warm, tingling feeling in your breasts that occurs shortly after your baby starts to suckle. The blood supply to your breasts also increases, with the supply that nourished the placenta being rerouted shortly after the birth. This is partly responsible for the engorgement and soreness that occurs in those early postpartum days.

DO I NEED TO PREPARE MY BREASTS?

In the past, women gave no thought to preparing their breasts for nursing. They either went bare-breasted or wore clothing that constantly rubbed against their unrestrained nipples. Nipple tissue that is constantly exposed to fresh air and sunlight and is unfettered by a bra is a lot more robust than if it's protected from the elements and from constant friction.

If you've always favoured an all-over suntan or burned your bra long ago, then your breasts are probably pretty well prepared for breast-feeding. Otherwise, if you'd like to do something in the way of preparing them, you can try moderate exposure to sunlight—just start off with very small doses and avoid exposure during the hottest part of the day. Since your breasts will be increasing in size, you may not be comfortable without a bra, so rubbing your nipples with a very soft towel after your shower can substitute for going bra-less. However if you've ever had a miscarriage (or even a threatened one), this gentle friction treatment is contraindicated, so just stick to fresh air and sunshine.

Zinc is involved in the formation of collagen, so adequate zinc status is important for ensuring the integrity of sensitive nipple tissue. The zinc taste test (see Chapter 5) can be applied at two-monthly intervals throughout your pregnancy and during breastfeeding, and you should supplement appropriately according to your zinc status. Soaps and shampoos can dry the natural oils secreted by your nipples, so avoid excessive contact with either.

You can also prepare your breasts by massaging them. Your partner might like to help! Use almond or apricot kernel oil, squeezing all around the areola in a scissoring motion, then pull out your nipples, rolling them gently between your thumb and forefinger to accustom them to being handled. Colostrum may be secreted when you do this. Just rub it into the nipple tissue—it has a protective effect.

A BETTER BIRTH AND BONDING MEANS BETTER BREASTFEEDING

A natural, unmedicated birth, unlimited skin-to-skin contact, the freedom for you to explore your baby's body, for your baby to come to your breast in his own time and for the bonding between you to take place without interruption will all ensure a wonderful start for a trouble-free and continuing breastfeeding relationship. Following your maternal instinct is easier too when you and your baby have this sort of beginning. If you're still pregnant (or even better, if you haven't conceived yet) and you want to give yourself the best possible chance of having a birth and bonding like this, and consequently a better breastfeeding experience, we recommend that you read all our earlier books.

Many of the medical procedures that accompany an assisted delivery are responsible for interrupted bonding and a difficult start to a breast-feeding relationship. Also, if you and your baby must be separated for any reason, or if there are attempts to limit the timing or duration of feeds in the early days, breastfeeding will be off to a less than ideal start. If you've already given birth and had the experience of bonding late or inappropriately, then you may be experiencing problems with breast-feeding, but don't despair. There's a lot that you can do to redress the balance.

CORRECT POSITIONING IS VITAL

A newborn baby who has had a completely natural birth, and is then simply placed on his mother's belly, will, within 50 minutes of the birth, make his way without any assistance whatever to the nipple and latch on. This instinctive response is achieved using the same pushing reflex that has propelled the baby from his mother's body, and always results in correct attachment to the nipple.

Take it slowly

Since incorrect attachment is one of the major causes of nipple trauma, it's important that you allow your baby to go to the breast at his own pace. If he's sleepy, as he will be after a medicated birth, just wait until he is awake and alert. Even though his sucking reflex is strongest in the first hour after birth, his ability to get it right if not hurried lasts for several weeks. Therefore it's important that you don't force your baby and also that you're not rushed and stressed yourself. If you take the time to sit quietly and let your baby latch on in his own time, you'll facilitate the correct attachment. Being relaxed and unhurried also promotes your let-down reflex. This will continue to be true for all your feeds—many babies like to lick, smell and mouth the nipple area before attaching, and these pre-feeding rituals will become a treasured part of your breast-feeding experience.

Encourage proper attachment

Hold your baby in the *en face* position, supporting him behind his neck and shoulders, not his head. A baby's natural response to having his head held is to push back against your hand, away from your breast. Bring him close in against you, so that his chin rests against the underneath part of your breast. Now point his nose towards your nipple so that he extends his head slightly, lifting his chin as he does so. His chin should be well in against your breast, with his nose clear so he can breathe easily. 'Chest to chest, chin to breast' is the motto. Then, with his chin tilted and his mouth fully open, he can take equal amounts of the top and bottom sections of the areola into his mouth, where they are held by suction. Equal pressure is important since it's the compression of the sinuses beneath the areola that causes the milk to be expelled through the nipple (which is merely a conduit). The nipple itself should not be grasped at all, but should move freely inside your baby's mouth. To understand how this works, suck your thumb and wiggle the end of it about in your mouth.

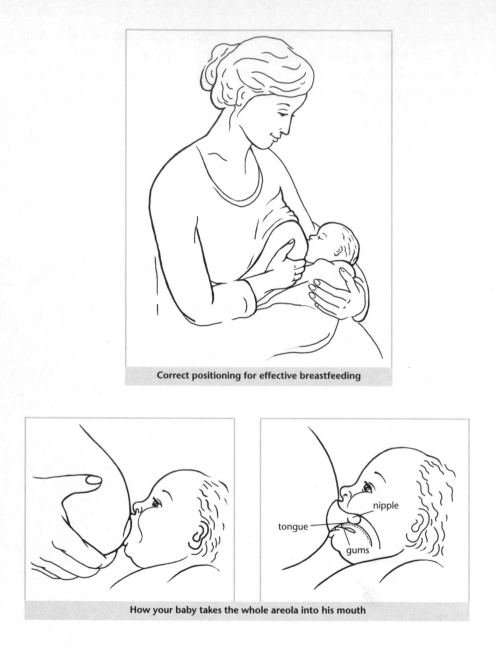

Correct positioning for effective breastfeeding

How your baby takes the whole areola into his mouth

If your baby has any difficulty finding your nipple, stroke his cheek nearest to your breast so he knows which way to face, and gently touch his mouth with your breast to encourage him to open his mouth wide and 'root' for your nipple. Have your nipple ready for that critical moment when he purses his lips in anticipation.

As your baby feeds he needs to have his body and head in a straight line to be comfortable, with his head slightly higher than his body to allow any air swallowed with the milk to come up easily. If he is lying on his back, he has to turn his head to reach your nipple. This makes swallowing difficult and he'll fight your breast. This is what causes nipple damage.

Clothes get in the way

It's best if you're both naked, especially in the early days. You'll get that vital skin-to-skin contact, and just as importantly for beginners you won't have to worry about trying to keep your shirt and bra and your baby's garments out of your way while you concentrate on correct positioning and attachment. If you can't manage to be naked when you're feeding, at least make sure your clothes are loose and that your baby can get at your breast easily. Also make sure that his clothing is uncluttered and comfortable. Avoid garments with buttons, bows and frills, and don't try to feed him while he's wrapped tightly in a shawl—not only will he be uncomfortable, but he may also be too hot. If he's too hot (or too cold) he won't be relaxed, and won't feed easily.

Be relaxed and comfortable

Comfort is really important for both of you, and finding the right position may need a little experimentation. If your baby lies across your lap, on his side, he will be facing you, and fulfilling the requirements we've just discussed. You will also be able to watch his face and look into his eyes as he feeds. However, if you need to hold your breast while nursing, you may find that having your baby on your lap causes you to twist your body and make you tense and sore, so it may be easier to tuck him under your arm, freeing up your other arm to reach across to hold your breast.

If you don't want to sit (for example when feeding in bed), lying on your side facing your baby will work well for both of you. When you are sitting, make sure you're in a chair with good back support, and don't hunch forward to reach your baby. 'Bring the baby to the breast, not the breast to the baby' is another useful reminder. You may need to put a cushion under him, to bring him up to where your breasts naturally hang. Old fashioned nursing chairs are low, without arms, to make it easier to sit with both feet flat on the floor and your back well supported.

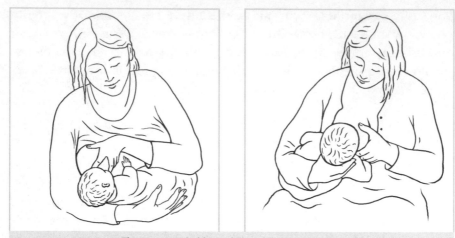

Three ways to hold your baby while breastfeeding

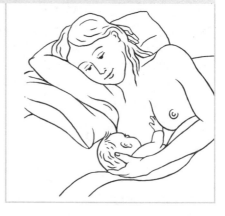

If you don't have one, you might find a footstool helpful, or you could try sitting cross-legged on the floor, with your back against the wall.

In order for you both to relax, it's best if you can feed in a place where you have privacy, peace and quiet, especially when your baby is very new and the feeding pattern is being established. You may find some soft lights and relaxing music helpful, and it'll be easier if there are no interruptions or time limits, though this may not always be in your control. You may get quite thirsty, and want to have some water or herbal tea at hand, so you can drink while he's feeding. If you're feeling jumpy, your baby will also be unsettled, so you should try to let go of any worries and anxieties and just enjoy the experience of nurturing your child. There are some ideas for relaxation and visualisation in Chapter 4, which you may find helpful.

Signs that all is well

Breastfeeding should not be uncomfortable or painful; it should feel delightful. When your baby's feeding well, his jaws, facial muscles and even the tips of his ears will all move. The wiggling-ear test is the best way to tell that he's feeding well. Although you may hear him swallow, loud tongue clicks or cheeks which hollow with each suck mean he isn't positioned properly. If it doesn't feel right for you, or he's uncomfortable, stop feeding and start again rather than persist in the wrong position, which will establish poor feeding patterns.

GET STARTED WITH SMALL, FREQUENT FEEDS

Feeding your baby frequently and for shorter periods in the days before your breasts become accustomed to breastfeeding can protect them from damage. This may require that you nurse your baby when you could otherwise settle him by rocking or patting. Letting your baby feed frequently also stimulates the hormones that promote lactation and ensures that they circulate freely through your blood supply. Oxytocin levels in your baby's brain are raised in response to the touch of his mouth on your nipple. This stimulates the release of 19 different gastrointestinal hormones that improve nutrient absorption. Oxytocin, released at let-down, also raises your pain threshold, creates slight drowsiness and euphoria and invokes a feeling of 'falling in love'. Endorphins, too, are produced during breastfeeding—these are natural mood enhancers and they further heighten the feelings of pleasure that you get when your baby nurses. So the more often you feed, the better you feel, the stronger the bond with your baby becomes, and the more familiar you become with the experience of nursing.

FORGET THE SCHEDULED FEEDS

As we've already mentioned, the scheduled feeding of infants has only been around for a couple of hundred years. Limiting the duration and number of feeds is a legacy of the intervention by scientifically orientated males in business that women had previously conducted intuitively. Sadly, the legacy of these men has been slow to die out. Even now, when we know that a healthy alert newborn may feed as many as sixteen or twenty times in 24 hours, many health professionals still advise three- or four-hourly feeds. If you're being pushed by a professional towards scheduled feeds, remember that babies *need* to feed often. The biology of human milk reflects the needs of the infant. The milk for a 'carrying' species is low in kilojoules. This translates into short feeding intervals. In carrying species, the infant is attached to the mother's body at all times and is therefore free to feed ad lib. Carrying species include apes and, in all earlier societies, humans. Conversely, milk for 'caches' species, such as ungulates (cattle, deer etc), is high in kilojoules. This translates into much longer feeding intervals because the baby, able to walk from just hours after the birth, can wander away from its mother between feeds.

But an infant who feeds at very short intervals is not what most of us expect or (frequently) want. Our cultural expectations are very well entrenched and our contemporary environment is not well suited to babies who sleep in short snatches and feed at frequent intervals. Infants who behave in this fashion are in defiance of the almost mythical (and much less well-adapted) babies who sleep soundly for three or four hours between feeds that take fewer than twenty minutes. We therefore become frustrated and look for the magic bullet to get our babies to adopt what we consider 'more appropriate' behaviour. However the problem doesn't lie with our babies, but with the fact that their biological needs and our present expectations and modern environment are badly mismatched. When you're a new mother and surrounded by other mothers who have a baby who is on a four-hourly schedule it's easy to feel that you're doing something wrong. We want to reassure you that you're actually doing something right when you ignore the advice from all quarters to get your baby to feed to a timetable.

The damage that timed and scheduled feeding does to the relationship between mother and baby is incalculable and the cases of early weaning that occur because of such restrictions are too numerous to contemplate. The cycle goes like this . . . Your baby cries. You don't believe he could possibly be hungry because you fed him only an hour ago. You forget that he may only want comfort, or that he may be trying to improve your milk supply or that he may actually be hungry or thirsty. You start to wonder if your milk is good enough. Your stress levels rise, causing prolactin levels to fall. This means that your milk supply diminishes. Your baby, breastfed less often than his needs dictate, fails to increase your milk supply. Consequently his hunger isn't satisfied, so he cries some more and the vicious cycle repeats itself.

Unfortunately, our advice to feed freely and often flies in the face of all those 'experts' who believe you just need to get your baby into a routine. A routine means that you feed him, wrap him firmly, put him down to settle and then he sleeps for hours. Of course lots of babies respond to this treatment, but many more don't for the reasons outlined above. Indeed, if you've got a 'better' baby, then you should be prepared for him to be very wakeful. When he's very young, all your baby wants during those wakeful periods is the comfort of your breast.

ONE BREAST OR TWO?

Don't feel you have to be bound by rules on whether to let your baby feed from one breast or two. However, if you let him completely empty a breast before moving on to the other one, he will get the fatty hindmilk, which will help him to feel more satisfied. The foremilk is more like a drink for him, whereas the hindmilk is the real meal. Also your body needs a clear message that it needs to produce an entire breastful, and that a half-full breast is just not good enough.

It depends on your baby's hunger, and how much milk you have, as to whether he will take one or both breasts at each feed, and this may vary. He'll let you know quite clearly when he's had enough—and when he wants more. However, if only one breast is emptied at a feed, make sure you offer the other breast next time. Put a breastpad in your bra on that side (you may well need it), or attach a safety pin to remind you to start with that breast at the next feed. Of course you may need no reminder; it may well be bursting with milk. Part of the pleasure of feeding is the release of the milk from a full breast.

DETACH HIM GENTLY

Babies' feeding patterns are as individual as the babies themselves. Some will be satisfied with brief periods of nursing while others seem to need almost constant oral gratification. If you have one of the latter, the frequent and lengthy nursing will often persist through periods of light sleep. As the baby falls asleep at your breast, the nipple slips from his mouth, upon which he rouses himself to continue sucking. It's often difficult to extract yourself from this limpet-like infant. If your frustration starts to get the better of you, or if you simply have to terminate the feed, it's important that you don't pull the nipple from your baby's mouth. Insert your finger between your baby's lips and your breast; this breaks the vacuum that his sucking has created and allows you to ease your nipple away from him.

CARRY YOUR BABY CLOSE

Carrying your baby close for as much of the day as you can is a great way to foster bonding and an easy breastfeeding relationship. (We'll look at what to do in the night-time hours in the next chapter.) It's also a great way to re-establish the closeness that you may have missed in the early hours, days or weeks following a less than ideal birth experience. Also, when you're carrying your baby in some sort of pouch or sling, you'll unconsciously touch his face, hold his hands, stroke his head and caress his body. It's a very simple way to satisfy a baby's fundamental biological need to be touched.

When you carry your baby like this you're simply repeating what mothers have done for thousands of years. Different forms of baby-carrying devices are as old as archaeological records, but putting babies into some sort of wheeled carriage or cot or basket is an extremely recent innovation. It's not surprising that very premature babies (who should still be in the womb) fare better if they're given 'kangaroo care'. Carried close at all times, with constant skin-to-skin contact, these tiny babies have a 60–90 per cent greater survival rate than those receiving orthodox intensive care.

When you carry your baby close, you'll become much more attuned to his rhythms of feeding and sleeping. If he's in your arms you'll know when he's ready to suck. Once you get the knack of feeding your baby while he's nestled in his sling, he'll probably feed frequently and sleep for short spells of about 20 minutes. The patterns of sleeping and eating, a preoccupation of the mothers of babies put down to sleep and picked up when crying, won't bother you at all.

Massage for bonding

As well as carrying him close, learning some simple techniques of baby massage can help you to connect and bond with your baby. If you're a bonded mother, you're more likely to be a breastfeeding mother. Mothers in traditional societies massage their babies regularly from birth. When you massage, you'll be able to feel and see your baby physically relax. What you cannot feel or see is his brain becoming denser—the cerebral cortex actually becomes heavier with this sort of stimulation. Your baby will also sense the warmth and caring imparted by your hands and will be much better able to return the nurturing when he's old enough.

FORGET THE DUMMY

The comfort and caring a baby needs certainly isn't provided by a dummy. Not only are bits of inert plastic or rubber shaped to resemble your nipple no substitute for the warmth and nurturing of the real thing, there are other valid reasons for avoiding them. If your baby is trying to build up your milk supply, using a dummy will thwart his attempts. If you use a dummy as a pacifier during the night, breastfeeding is unlikely to provide a contraceptive effect. Babies are less likely to grow out of needing to suck on a dummy than on a thumb or finger, and may continue to be attached to it long after sucking is appropriate or healthy. Using a dummy may lead to 'nipple confusion'. Since the placement of the tongue during breastfeeding is different from when a teat or dummy is sucked, dummies can encourage incorrect attachment. Finally, studies show that women who give their baby a dummy breastfeed for shorter periods than those women who use their breast as a pacifier.

GIVE YOUR BABY TIME TO NURSE

As your baby grows, his breastfeeding experiences become increasingly marked by pauses and non-verbal interactions. This can be a frustrating experience if you view these distractions as detracting from the 'real' purpose of nursing—simply satisfying hunger and thirst. However if you think of them as akin to having a good meal with a fine bottle of wine, enjoyed and savoured with a lover or cherished friend, you have a better idea of what your baby is getting at your breast.

The distractions—as he plays with your clothes, strokes your skin, fiddles with your other nipple—and the pauses—when he looks around, gazes up at you, then resumes—are the beginnings of his social interactions. Take the time to foster them. What is taking place is a sophisticated, non-verbal dialogue. It is the beginning of language. By allowing the time for these interactions to play out (no matter how much you wish your baby would just get on with his business, letting you get on with yours), you are acknowledging his importance as a person and, believe it or not, establishing clear communication channels for the future. So give your baby plenty of time to nurse, stop, interact, nurse again, pause, fiddle and nurse some more. You're enhancing his development into a socially adept human being.

WHAT IF BREASTFEEDING ISN'T EASY?

Sometimes, despite your best intentions, you and your baby may not get the hang of breastfeeding straight away. If that happens (and even if it doesn't), you'll find that just about everyone with whom you come in contact in the days when you're trying to establish your breastfeeding relationship will have some advice to offer. While this advice may be very well intentioned, it may also be contradictory and sometimes it can be downright unhelpful, as we've already seen.

Consult a real expert

Rather than rely on the offerings of enthusiastic amateurs (or less than well-qualified health professionals), get advice from an appropriately trained practitioner if you're having problems of any kind. An experienced lactation consultant is undoubtedly the best person to help you, since she will be totally committed to a continuing breastfeeding relationship. If any other so-called experts offer advice that casts doubt on your ability to breastfeed, be it for reasons of skin or hair colour, nipple or breast size or shape, genetics, your own or your family history, your baby's physical condition or growth patterns or the abundance or otherwise of your milk supply, always get a second opinion from a lactation consultant.

Support groups can help

If you're not experiencing any particular problems, or if you're simply hoping to avoid them, we recommend that you join a support group. Once, all women were well acquainted with the mechanics of breastfeeding before they had their own child. They almost certainly had the opportunity to learn about it at the optimum time, which is at three, four or five years of age, when they simply saw it happening all around them. But as the rate of breastfeeding declines, as the length of time for which women feed their children gets shorter and as the number of children in a family also falls, there are fewer and fewer opportunities for learning in this way.

For most women today breastfeeding is an art that must be learned, and watching other women breastfeed is still the best way to do it. If you can manage it, the very best time to learn (as it always has been) is long before you hold your baby in your arms.

Meetings are held regularly and mothers interact and encourage one another in an informal setting (usually one of the mothers' homes). Watching other mothers breastfeed can affirm your belief that this is a natural, uncomplicated activity and also that breastfeeding is not just for babies. These get-togethers may also provide more than a source of information on breastfeeding matters. They can be a valuable reference point on all topics related to raising children. Today, when many women live far from their mothers and sisters, these groups can provide encouragement and support for the woman who is doing something that she once would have done without even thinking. Also, the groups offer 24-hour emergency services, with trained breastfeeding counsellors available to give help with any problems that crop up.

Books can help

Books can also provide a great deal of valuable information, but as with 'expert' advice make sure that the book you choose is one that favours a natural approach rather than recommending scheduled feeds and 'controlled crying'. We give some suggestions for appropriate reading material in the Recommended Reading section. Of course the book you're holding in your hands is as good as you'll get for the natural approach, but sometimes you might want some reinforcement!

CARE OF YOUR BREASTS

Of course to ensure the success of a long-term breastfeeding relationship you'll need to take good care of your breasts. Wear a good, comfortable maternity bra and use a nursing pad inside the cup if your breasts leak. The pad should be changed frequently; try not to leave a wet pad in contact with your breast for too long. Your nipples should be kept clean and dry. As we've already mentioned, it's better not to use soap on your nipples—it takes the fat out of the tissue and you'll be more prone to cracks and sores. When you dry your breasts, patting may be preferable to rubbing if they tend to be sore. Also, if you can, leave your bra off after feeding so your nipples get an airing whenever possible.

As well as zinc, which we mentioned earlier, other nutrient minerals important for healthy breasts are selenium (best as seleno-methionine), magnesium, manganese and calcium. The essential fatty acids (from Evening Primrose and fish oils) and Garlic are helpful for healthy breasts, as are vitamins A, B-complex, C and E. Of the B-complex vitamins, B1, B3 and B6 are particularly indicated, but refer to Chapter 5 for more on dosage of vitamin B6. Check carefully that garlic isn't upsetting to your baby; his bowel movements will let you know if it is causing him problems.

Vegetable juices are a great source of helpful nutrients, and you need plenty of fluids to keep your breasts functioning well. Coffee, cigarettes and alcohol are particularly harmful, as are heavy metals, since all these toxins will accumulate in the fatty tissue of your breasts. See Chapter 6 for advice on keeping your breast milk safe; if you follow it you'll also protect your breasts from harm.

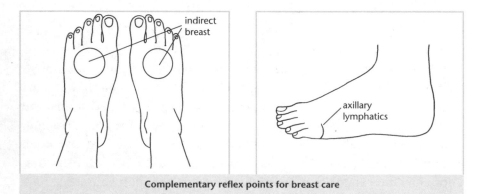

Complementary reflex points for breast care

Additionally, there are some reflexology points and zones you can use for general preventative care of your breasts. As well as the points suggested on p. 65 for improving your milk supply, you can also use the complementary zones: the indirect breast zone on the top of your feet, and the axillary lymphatics zone shown above. Massage of the whole breast area can also help to keep them healthy. There's more on how to use reflexology in Appendix 5, and in Chapter 10 there's detailed information on how to cope with the physical problems that may arise even in the best breastfeeding relationships (though if you follow our advice they should be less likely to crop up). Let's look now though at an issue that unnecessarily disturbs many new mothers—whether they have sufficient milk to feed their babies.

Making sure you have plenty of milk

As we pointed out in the previous chapter, the more frequently you feed your baby, the more milk you produce. This elegant rule of supply and demand ensures that if you feed your baby as often as he needs, you'll always have enough milk to satisfy him. So when your baby goes through periods of wanting to feed every hour or two (or even more frequently), just hang in there. Don't be concerned that he isn't satisfied; he's probably just trying to boost your milk supply.

This increased frequency of feeding usually happens during periods of very rapid growth that occur at around 5–6 weeks and again at 3–6 months. Some babies also have a growth spurt about three weeks after the birth, and increased frequency of feeds may also occur if your baby is sick or teething. Of course, if you doubt this rule and introduce supplementary feeds of any sort, your own supply will certainly diminish because your baby will nurse less frequently. Giving water is also counter-productive. Babies who are fully breastfed do not need supplementary water, even in the very hottest weather.

If you're concerned about your ability to satisfy your baby and in doubt about whether he's getting enough, you might wish that your breasts were transparent and clearly calibrated so that you could see how much milk your baby takes at a feed. Thankfully your breasts are a lot more attractive than a plastic bottle or measuring jug, but to allay any concerns there are some very obvious physical markers that clearly indicate whether your baby is getting enough.

IS HE GETTING ENOUGH?

Don't assume that because your baby cries, he is hungry and you haven't enough milk; there are lots of reasons why he may cry (see Chapter 11). Also don't worry that your milk looks thin or blue compared to cow's milk, as this is quite normal. It may look particularly thin in the evening if you're over-tired or haven't eaten well, as the fat content may be lowered. To be sure of maintaining good quality milk well into the evening, with a high fat content which helps to make your baby sleepy, make sure you eat well through the day—a good lunch is the most important meal. Also, don't worry if your breasts seem small or not full. This is not necessarily any indication of milk supply.

An adequate weight gain (500 grams a month or more) indicates that your breast milk is providing everything your baby needs. However, it's worth remembering that a lot of the age–weight charts are still based on the weight gain of bottle-fed babies, and that bottle-fed babies grow much faster than those that are breastfed, simply because cow's milk formula is based on a product that was designed for the rapid weight gain of calves! Other indicators, that are just as important, are good muscle tone, bright eyes, a strong cry and a baby who is alert when awake and content after a feed. Finally, if your baby produces six to eight wet nappies every day, then he is certainly getting enough from your breast.

But if his urine is bright yellow with a strong smell or he urinates fewer than six times a day; if he has infrequent, small, hard, dry or green stools; if the fontanelle (the soft spot on his forehead) is sunken or if he becomes very quiet and listless, then he definitely needs more breast milk—and needs it fast. Feed freely and often if any of these signs are present. A breastfeed every two or three hours (or more often) during a 24-hour period should do the trick. If you feed your baby at every opportunity and he still doesn't seem to gain much weight or if other markers indicate that your supply isn't as good as it should be, we've got some other ideas for how to improve it. Of course, if your baby is exhibiting serious symptoms like those described just above, and he does not respond well within twenty-four hours, you should seek prompt medical advice.

IMPROVING YOUR SUPPLY OF MILK

Relax

Stress inhibits the production of prolactin. When prolactin levels fall, your milk supply diminishes. So forget about the housework for a while. If you can't bear the dust, the unwashed dishes and the mounting pile of laundry, and find ignoring the mess as stressful as trying to clean it up, enlist some help. Ask your partner to take over the running of the house for a while. He might not do it quite the way you would, but he might also surprise you with his ability. Ask a relative or friend to stay for a week or two. As long as you get on well and there's enough room, it can be a Godsend to have an extra pair of hands around. Ask a favour if someone drops by. True friends respond well to being asked to hang out a load of laundry or cook a pot of soup. Don't try to be superwoman. Nursing your baby is your primary concern for the moment and in the early weeks it's a fulltime job.

As your baby starts to grow and your breastfeeding relationship becomes more established and familiar, you'll feel a lot less stressed if you make sure you get some time to yourself occasionally. Babysitting by your partner, your family or friends can be easily achieved if you express some milk in advance (see p. 52). (Leaving a bottle of formula for the babysitter defeats the whole purpose of the exercise.) Then you can indulge in some exercise (see Chapter 7), which is excellent for stress management, or some activity to stimulate the old grey matter. The first few months may not be the best time to take up studying for a degree; apart from the extra demands on your time which you need to accommodate, Mother Nature has a neat trick up her sleeve to stop you focusing on anything too strenuous. Studies bear out the popular belief that women become more forgetful in those first few postnatal months, and you may find that remembering all your new domestic duties is quite enough to cope with. Although this may be contrary to your 'girls can do anything' philosophy, remember 'anything' includes having babies—a very important job. A fun recreational course, however, may be just what you need to stimulate the brain and give you some time to yourself.

EXPRESSING MILK

Expressing milk ensures that your baby has access to a supply of breast milk if you need to be away from him or are too ill to feed him. It can be important in maintaining his good health if you need time out to recover yours (see Chapter 10 for how to cope if you are ill). It may also be necessary if you need to leave him with someone else on occasion, and can provide an opportunity for his father to feed him and enjoy the closeness of that experience. You may also need to express between feeds if you have too much milk, or if it's too long between feeds, especially if only one breast is emptied at each feed.

HOW TO EXPRESS

There are many different types of breast pump, and all come with full instructions (see Contacts and Resources), but if you're likely to need a substantial supply of expressed milk you might consider hiring an electric pump. If you're expressing for relief, you'll be able to express by hand: just gently squeeze your breast towards the nipple. If you do this under a hot shower the milk will flow more easily.

Expressing whenever you eat or drink (eight times in 24 hours) will maintain your supply and ensure plenty for your baby. If you're trying to boost your supply, make sure that you express during the night as well. Expressed breast milk will keep in the fridge for up to 24 hours, or can be frozen and stored for up to 3 months in a deep freeze or for up to 2 weeks in the freezer compartment of your fridge. Use it within 12 hours of defrosting. It should be stored in sterilised containers (your chemist can supply bags specially designed for this purpose) and your breast pump should also be sterilised after each use.

HOW TO FEED YOUR BABY EXPRESSED MILK

It's preferable not to give your baby expressed milk through a bottle, as the way he sucks on the teat is different from the action at the breast, and he will learn poor habits. If you do need to use a bottle, make sure you acquire a long latex teat, which mimics a nipple more closely than one made of silicone.

Alternative ways of feeding include via a spoon or a cup. If you're using a cup, hold your baby in a semi-upright position and rest a small cup or glass on his bottom lip, tipping it so a few drops run into his mouth. He will soon learn to lap the milk from the edge of the cup. Don't put too much milk in the cup at any one time. If you're using a spoon use a similar action, tipping the spoon slowly.

One of the nicest ways to spend your time to yourself is to pay some attention to your appearance and buy some new clothes or maybe get your hair styled or have a facial. Looking good lifts your spirits and that helps you to be more relaxed.

One of the joys of breastfeeding, however, is that your baby is portable. Or rather your breasts are. A bottle-fed baby has to go everywhere accompanied by essential paraphernalia, but your baby just needs you. So don't think that relaxation means staying at home permanently. While frenetic activity is the last thing we'd advocate, especially in the early weeks or months, staying at home 24 hours a day can also be very stressful.

Although visitors can be another welcome distraction, especially if you're used to the companionship of the workplace, don't overdo the hospitality at first. Especially discourage endless strange faces oohing and aahing at your baby—an overstimulated baby won't feed well and will get jittery.

You may find it stressful when your baby cries; we'll look at some of the reasons and remedies for this in Chapter 11. You may also find it hard when he's at his most wakeful, and you're not. Babies are often most wide awake in the evenings, between five and nine or ten o'clock—just when you may need some recovery time. We suggest that the best way to deal with this is to include your baby in your family activities at this time; that'll keep him interested and cheerful. If you try to put him to sleep in order to have an 'adult' evening you'll just end up frustrated and upset (and so will he).

If you're concerned about the effect that all your attention on your new baby may have on older siblings, get them to do something special at breastfeeding time, with their father perhaps, that's a treat reserved for those occasions.

If you feel exhausted, or you just need to be quiet, take the phone off the hook (or put on the answering machine), and practise some of the following ways to relax. If you feel that your emotional state is verging on postnatal depression—if you're tearful, fearful, over-irritable or just plain depressed—either seek professional help or at least see our previous book, *Healthy Body, Better Birthing*, for more suggestions.

Aids to relaxation

Herbal teas

There are lots of ways to help yourself relax. Herbal teas such as Chamomile, Catnip, Hops and Lemon Balm can gently soothe you, and help you to sleep. You can make a herbal infusion (see instructions in Appendix 5) or you can acquire a stronger fluid extract form from a herbalist, who may combine it with adaptogens, remedies which support your adrenals and your energy levels. Herbs that you can use in this way include Withania and Siberian Ginseng. If you eat plenty of porridge or muesli, you'll get a good supply of Oats, an excellent nerve tonic. Small amounts of these remedies (just enough for a small body) will filter through your breast milk to your baby, helping him to calm down too.

Flower essences

Flower essences that act gently on emotional states which can be helpful for new mothers include Bottlebrush and Walnut to help you deal with change and outside influences, Bush Fuchsia to help you trust your intuition, Vervain to calm you, Olive and Hornbeam to help with low energy states, Larch to help you overcome lack of confidence, and Gentian for discouragement. Black-eyed Susan or Impatiens are for those times when you're feeling irritable, rushed or frustrated, Red Chestnut for overconcern for others (maybe your baby or partner), Oak for struggling on through despondency, and Mustard for depression and gloom. Flower essences are completely non-toxic and safe to use during breastfeeding; just take a few drops under your tongue several times a day.

Aromatherapy and massage

Aromatherapy can be an enjoyable way to relieve stress. Essential oils such as Lavender can be used in a massage, sprinkled on your pillow or in your bath, or heated in an oil burner. One oil to avoid is Jasmine which can suppress breast milk through its action on prolactin. Essential oils should not be used on your baby or in his bath. Massage, of course, can be helpful for relaxation even without essential oils; this would be a great treat to give yourself occasionally. Your partner may be able to oblige, if not with the massage, then with the baby-sitting!

Relaxation therapy

When the term 'relaxation therapy' is used, it usually refers to some form of guided visualisation, meditation or hypnotherapy. Studies have shown a link between the use of such therapies and a reduction in allergic response in the children of breastfeeding mothers. We'd like to offer you here an easy relaxation exercise which you can do while you're breast-feeding, if you need to calm down. Unlike most relaxation sessions, you probably won't want to close your eyes, because nursing is the time you are closest to your child. It'll also be easier if any pictures you imagine are related to the activity of feeding, so you are able to enter into it more fully, rather than drifting off somewhere else.

It's very simple to just direct your breath to each part of your body— one breath at a time—and feel the tensions drain away. Start with your feet and work up your body via your back, shoulders, neck and head, then bring the focus of your attention back to your breasts. Imagine you can see the milk forming and flowing, like a river of life, glowing with energy. You can then watch as your baby fills out and starts to glow himself. Believe us, this really does happen at feeding time, even without your dreaming.

Another similar calming technique is to use an affirmation, or mantra, to dispel distractions or anxiety. Here are some suggestions.

'I have all the time in the world to nurture my baby.'

'This is the time I share with my child.'

'I am centred here, and now, with my baby.'

'Feeding my baby brings us both joy.'

'When I'm feeding my child, time stands still.'

Of course, as you relax, so does your baby and that, in its turn, will help you to stay calm.

Get enough sleep

Sleeping with your baby beside you is the easiest way to get enough sleep, and it's best for baby too. Sharing your bed is undoubtedly the simplest solution to attending to the baby who wakes for feeds during the night. Yet, the very mention of communal sleeping quarters brings up doubts and fears in many parents. Couples who take their child into their bed often do so reluctantly and as a last (rather than a first) resort. They fear that they might smother their baby, they are uncertain about possible sexual deviation precipitated by co-sleeping and are very concerned about what friends and relatives will say. They worry that co-sleeping will rupture their conjugal relationship and encourage their child to be excessively dependent. They wonder whether a child allowed into the parental bed will ever want to leave it. But if parents thought logically and calmly, they would realise that the family bed or co-sleeping is not a radical or trendy parenting alternative. It is simply sleeping in the same way that the human species has slept for more than 99.99 per cent of its time on this planet. For countless centuries, for countless families in countless countries, the family bed was simply the only way of sleeping. In other words, solitary sleeping arrangements for infants (and for adults as well) have been around for only about as long as the blink of an eye in evolutionary terms.

So perhaps we should pay some attention to what we are doing when we force children to sleep alone. Perhaps we should not accept separate sleeping arrangements for all family members as the norm. James McKenna, Professor of Biological Anthropology and Director of the Mother–Baby Behavioural Sleep Laboratory at the University of Notre Dame USA, has this to say. 'Solitary sleeping arrangements represent one of the least recognised, but certainly one of the most potentially significant cultural experiments of the nineteenth and twentieth centuries, the consequences of which have never been scientifically explored.'

Indeed, there is not one scientific study that documents the deleterious consequences of co-sleeping or the benefits of solitary sleeping. Rather, studies show that there are positive benefits to be had when a family shares its sleeping quarters.

Benefits of co-sleeping

Convenience and reduced stress
The brain of your newborn baby is still immature. In the early months of his life he will experience long periods of sleep from which he can be easily aroused. This means he will wake fairly frequently. This sleep pattern, which is unique to infants, is thought to be important for brain development. Since that development continues rapidly until about three years of age when the brain approaches 90 per cent of its adult capacity, it is unlikely that a healthy baby will sleep for an unbroken six or eight hours during the night.

It is also an unrealistic expectation that you will rouse yourself from deep sleep without complaint, rise from your warm bed and attend to your baby whenever he wakes. By giving your baby separate sleeping quarters, night-time becomes unnecessarily stressful and your baby is denied the things that he needs most—your warmth, the sound of your heartbeat, your touch and your milk.

FAMILY BED, FAMILY SIZE

Once you have a new baby in the family, the need for a family bed—one that will truly accommodate a family—is an absolute priority. The benefits of family sleeping are beyond question, but your bed needs to be spacious enough to accommodate the wriggling, sideways lying and frequent moves from one breast to the other that are features of your growing baby. All of this activity, and the chance that there may be more than one child in the bed as well, can make co-sleeping in a small, regulation size double bed a real endurance test. A king or queen size bed, or a low double bed with a small mattress (or mattresses) attached 'side-car' fashion, will give the whole family room to sleep in peace.

When you take your new baby into your bed, lie him down directly on the mattress; he doesn't need a pillow. Lie half on your side, enclosing him in the crook of your arm. Don't overdress him, because he'll absorb your body heat. Swap him to the opposite side after he's finished feeding so that he can root for your other nipple at the next feed. Once he can crawl, all of this becomes unnecessary, and often you'll wake wondering how he finished up where he is and how many times he nursed.

Synchronised sleep patterns

A nursing mother and her co-sleeping infant have synchronised sleep and arousal patterns. This arousal–sleep–arousal cycle, which lasts about ninety minutes in an adult, is also the usual length of time between feeds for the co-sleeping baby. When there is co-ordination of sleep cycles the mother enters the light phase of sleep, from which she is easily aroused, just as her baby wakes and begins to nurse. This means her sleep is less disturbed since she is already in the light sleep phase. Although the co-sleeping mother and baby are aroused more often than if they slept separately, their total sleep time is greater. Furthermore, co-sleeping mothers only remember about half of their baby's wakings and feedings.

Protection from SIDS and apnoea

The co-sleeping baby spends a greater length of time in light sleep and maintains this easy arousal when sleeping alone, which is an inherent safety factor for him. By contrast, the average sleep cycle of the solitary baby is about 200 minutes, and he spends a much greater length of time in deep sleep from which he is not easily aroused. The fact that co-sleeping babies spend less time in deep sleep and more time in the supine position (in order to feed) protects them from SIDS, as lying face down is now confirmed as a risk factor.

A co-sleeping baby also responds to his mother's breathing (or his father's) and his apnoea rate is reduced (apnoea is the cessation of breathing during sleep). The inhalation of carbon dioxide acts on the receptors in his brain, triggering the breathing response. All the mechanisms regulating respiratory rate, heart rate, oxygen saturation and other significant factors operate better when the baby is in direct contact with his mother. This doesn't happen by chance. There is a direct sensory exchange leading to a rise in the baby's axillary and skin temperature, an increase in blood glucose levels, preservation of glycogen stores and increased oxygen saturation.

Reduced crying

As a nursing mother and child enter the light phase of sleep together, the baby will stir and start to suckle. He won't cry, since the nipple is within reach of his mouth and his mother's sleep is only slightly disturbed as she becomes dimly aware of him nursing. Then both return to a state of deeper sleep. Some 20–40 per cent of babies will respond to separation from their parents by crying. With co-sleeping, crying is reduced in frequency and any crying periods are of short duration, nursing is well established earlier and the baby gains weight faster.

The contraceptive effect

Babies who routinely share the parental bed feed between two and three times as frequently and for up to three times as long as solitary sleepers. This increased frequency and duration of nursing means that prolactin levels remain high. This means that milk supply is enhanced and also that ovulation is suppressed. The fact that a mother is breastfeeding during the day is simply not enough to ensure a contraceptive effect. Rather it is the nature and structure of the feeds during the night that ensure lactational amenorrhoea. Suppressed ovulation ensures a longer interval between pregnancies and both the mother and the baby benefit nutritionally and emotionally from this enforced child spacing.

Mother and baby respond to each other
The co-sleeping mother responds to her baby in various subtle ways. She touches him, moves him, pulls up the covers, tucks him in, kisses him and cuddles him. The baby responds to the mother too and even in sleep he turns to face her nipple.

Sense of security
It's hardly surprising that a child who shares the family sleeping quarters is rarely reluctant to go to bed. He suffers much less frequently from nightmares and also has fewer fears and phobias than the child who sleeps alone. A co-sleeping child gets better faster when he is sick. He is a confident child and never knows the feeling of insecurity that can come from sleeping alone. His sense of 'rightness' and belonging has been fostered from his earliest days by co-sleeping.

Sense of rightness
You might wake to find a tiny mouth rooting for a nipple, or your toddler crawling over you to help himself from the other breast. You might simply wake and watch your baby sleeping peaceful and serene. Whatever it may be, there is a certain sense of rightness when you share your nights as well as your days with your child. If your partner does not see much of his child during the day, or if you need to go back to work, sharing a bed is an easy and wonderful way to redress some of this imbalance.

The easiest way to achieve minimal disturbance is for the whole family to sleep together. As well as being the only sane, sensible and easily workable solution to the reality of a baby who likes to feed, or needs to be comforted, on numerous occasions throughout the night, having your baby in bed with you is surely one of the great joys of parenthood.

But what about those negatives the proponents of solitary sleeping love to raise when you mention the family bed? Let's dispel some of the myths that have grown up around co-sleeping.

What happens to your sex life?

If you worry about your sex life, and this seems to be the stumbling block and major point of contention for many couples debating the merits of the family bed, rest assured that small children have shared parental beds for far longer than they have slept alone. They have also probably been dimly aware of what went on in that bed and developed far healthier attitudes to sex than many children have today. If you are unable to be uninhibited, you can at least be inventive and find somewhere else to make love.

You won't squash your baby

Unless you've been drinking or taking drugs, you'll be very aware of your baby's presence and in no danger of squashing or lying on him. However if you're the worrying kind and unlikely to sleep well because of your concern, a crib or mattress at your bedside is the answer.

One day he'll be gone!

You can rest assured that when your child feels secure and sure of his place in the family he will initiate a move to a bed of his own. If you are concerned that he will never be independent, you should remember that independence is achieved only when he is ready, and can't be rushed or forced. Until that time, simply foster your child's sense of security so that he can achieve true independence when the time is right for him.

Till then, your baby does not stop needing you when it gets dark. If he continues to wake through the night for months, or sometimes years, to come (as it seems that babies were designed to do) you will only maintain your equilibrium, your good humour and your sanity if your sleep is minimally disturbed.

While enough sleep during the night is vital if you're going to have an abundant supply of breast milk, don't forget that a daytime nap also works wonders for keeping stress levels down and milk supply up. With your baby sound asleep, it might seem like the ideal time to get on with all those undone chores, but forget them for the moment and lie down with your baby beside you instead!

All the remedies and techniques we've discussed for relaxation will be helpful to encourage good quality sleep, and you can find more in our previous books. Sleep deprivation can be a major problem for new mums, and you need to address it before it saps your energy and you go for the quick fixes of sugar or caffeine, which will only cause your baby to be restless and irritable, and compound your problem.

Stay well hydrated

Even when you're not breastfeeding, you need to drink at least 2 litres of purified water a day to stay well hydrated. While you're nursing, you'll need to increase that by 500 mL–1 litre daily, or more during very hot weather. Remember that your baby gets all the fluid he needs from your breasts and his needs will increase in hot weather just as yours do. Here are some other ideas for good drinking habits.

- Drinking fruit juice isn't a good idea as even unsweetened fruit juice contains a high load of fruit sugars. Soft drinks are definitely off the menu.

- Drinking cow's milk isn't recommended as it's a very common allergen. If anyone tries to tell you that it's necessary to boost your supply you might ask how a cow, consuming only grass, ever manages!

- Drink teas made from *Nettle*, *Alfalfa*, *Fenugreek*, *Fennel* (seeds), *Chamomile*, *Red Clover* and *Raspberry*. These teas are known to promote lactation and can be mixed together to produce a flavour which you find pleasant. So experiment with them. Of course, any of the herbs in our 'allowed' list in Appendix 2 can also be used. To get the full benefit of the herbs, leave them to infuse for at least 10–15 minutes (see Appendix 5). You can drink several cups a day of these gently acting herbs, but cut down if your breasts start to burst! Although black tea, which is naturally low in caffeine, is not likely to upset your baby, it is diuretic in its action so won't be helpful for hydration.

- Beer (or stout) has been traditionally drunk by breastfeeding mothers, but we don't recommend alcohol when you're breastfeeding. You could try *Hops*, however; this is what beer is made from and the reason that it's been useful to nursing mothers.

Eat well and take your supplements

This important subject is covered in detail in the next chapter, but we'll give you a brief overview here of foods especially good for promoting milk supply.

Especially helpful are wholegrains (particularly barley, oats and brown rice), leafy greens (Dandelion and Nettle can be included in your salads), apricots, asparagus, avocados, nuts (especially almonds), sea vegetables and red, orange and yellow vegetables. You can try juicing your vegetables (the nutrients are more readily available and you'll get more of them). Juicing is also a quick and easy alternative when you haven't got the time or energy to prepare a meal.

Add lots of Garlic to your food to promote lactation. Most babies like it, and two clinical trials have shown that garlic benefits both mother and baby. However, some babies are irritated by garlic and get loose stools, as they can with onions and chillies. Useful culinary herbs and spices include Coriander, Cumin, Caraway, Dill and Aniseed.

Adequate protein is very important as two of the amino acids which make up protein, phenylalanine and tyrosine, have a role in promoting lactation. Finally, as well as maintaining an excellent diet, you should take a comprehensive range of essential nutrients in supplement form for the whole period of breastfeeding.

Herbal and homoeopathic remedies

Some herbs are known to promote the flow of milk and are listed below. Many of them are also nutritive and help to replace minerals that may have become depleted during pregnancy and feeding. Most of them also have other therapeutic actions which are detailed in the list. Remember, your baby gets the benefit too, through the milk. Some of them can be found in your health food shop as dried herbs and used as a tea (see Appendix 5 for instructions on how to prepare teas). For a stronger action, the fluid extracts can be used, at a dosage set by a herbalist.

Choose from the following, if you're concerned about your milk supply:

- Alfalfa—helpful for acidity. As it contains phyto-oestrogens, be moderate in your intake, or reserve its use for times when your milk supply is threatened

- Aniseed—a carminative herb, which will aid digestion and reduce wind

- Catnip—an excellent nervine, especially recommended for children, also helpful for colic

- Chamomile—very calming to the nerves and the digestion

- Chastetree—although this herb, which acts on the pituitary gland, suppresses abnormally raised prolactin levels outside of lactation, while you are feeding it promotes milk production. It may be better to use a dose which is at the lower end of the therapeutic dosage range, which is more likely to increase prolactin levels. Be guided by a herbalist

- Dandelion—the root is an excellent liver tonic. Take care with the leaves, for though they are nutritive and promote milk production, they are also diuretic. Make sure you drink lots of water

- Dill—very helpful for colic

- Fennel—decreases colic in your baby. If taking this as a tea, the seeds are used, and you'll get more benefit if you crack them before infusing. This herb is also oestrogenic; see caution as for Alfalfa

- Fenugreek—helps to reduce catarrhal conditions

- Goat's Rue—helpful if you've had any blood sugar problems

- Hops—an excellent sedative

- Nettles—a wonderfully supportive herb for the kidneys and uterus, and very high in nutrients

- Raspberry—will help your uterus to recover after childbirth, and is highly nutritive

- Red Clover—a traditional blood cleanser or detoxifier. Contains phyto-oestrogens

Squaw Vine—a good general reproductive tonic. It can also be applied to nipples that are sore

St Mary's Thistle—very helpful for the liver and digestion

You can also try these homoeopathic remedies:

Pulsatilla—if there's poor supply due to stress and anxiety

Lac defloratum—if your milk dries up altogether

Homoeopathy is completely non-toxic and safe to use during breast-feeding, but can be quite powerful in its effect. The best results will be obtained if you consult a professional homoeopath. See Appendix 5 for more information on how to use homoeopathy.

Acupressure, massage and reflexology

For self-help, try the following recommended points. For more thorough treatment, visit a health professional. (See Appendix 5 for detailed instructions on how to apply acupressure.)

Try stimulating *Gall Bladder 21*, using tonifying pressure. To find this point, draw a straight line up from the nipple. The point is where it crosses the top of the shoulder

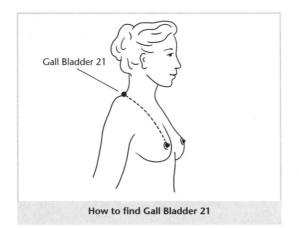

How to find Gall Bladder 21

❧ Massage the reflex zones for the breasts, hypothalamus and pituitary

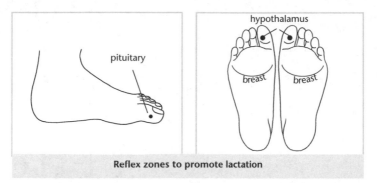

Reflex zones to promote lactation

❧ Gently massage your breasts with the palm of your hands, in a clockwise direction

So now you know how to ensure a plentiful supply of milk, let's look at what you can do to ensure that the milk you produce is of the very best quality. If you've read our earlier books, you'll already be familiar with the material in the next chapter, because, surprise, surprise, one of the most fundamental steps to achieving top quality breast milk—and breastfeeding success—is good nutrition!

Healthy eating for better breastfeeding

Healthy eating habits are something that we never tire of talking about, simply because they are at the basis of every stage of successful reproduction. So the best time to make the changes to your diet necessary for a successful breastfeeding relationship, and to begin a program of supplementation which will help to ensure it, is well before you actually conceive (read Healthy Parents, Better Babies for all the information). But if you didn't give your diet the attention it deserves before conception and during your pregnancy (see Healthy Lifestyle, Better Pregnancy and Healthy Body, Better Birthing), don't despair. It's certainly never too late, and whatever positive changes you make and whenever you make them will have benefits for both you and your baby. If you've read our previous books, you'll be familiar with much of the material that follows, since the guidelines for eating well while you're breastfeeding your baby are, not surprisingly, very close to those for when you're pregnant, about to give birth, or trying to conceive. So what are the particular benefits of good nutrition now that you've given birth to your baby?

WHY IS NUTRITION IMPORTANT FOR BREASTFEEDING?

That all-important factor—maternal instinct—depends on adequate supplies of all essential nutrients. So does the quality of your breast milk, particularly if the breastfeeding relationship is to be a long-term one. What's more, you can avoid postnatal depression, cracked nipples, an excessively crying baby and can also ensure that his demands don't cause the excessive fatigue that is a characteristic of early (and not so early) postpartum days, by eating and supplementing appropriately.

Even if you've been diligent about your diet and supplementation right up until the birth, good eating habits can fly out the window after your baby's born. Your new arrival takes up an enormous amount of your time in those early weeks and that's even more likely to be the case if it's your first baby. What's more, breastfeeding puts extra demands on your nutritional stores, so your appetite will increase after the birth. When you've got little time to prepare food, or when you have a ravenous appetite, it's easy to reach for the fast food, packaged, ready-to-hand options.

So we suggest that you stock up on healthy, easy-to-prepare food, or have some of your favourite recipes frozen for use during the early weeks of your baby's life. But it's not really enough to say eat well and stock your pantry and your freezer. We're now going to examine in detail why some nutrients are so important at this time, and we'll then discuss the best ways to go about getting them in the correct balance and combination.

NECESSARY NUTRIENTS

Zinc and manganese for maternal instinct

It might surprise you to learn that your nutritional status can affect something as fundamental as the instinctive desire to mother your baby. This desire is essential for your baby's wellbeing, and the trace element zinc is important to ensure that your mothering behaviour is appropriate. Animal studies have shown that zinc-deficient rat mothers build no nests, they don't nurse their young, won't retrieve the young that stray, and may even totally abandon their offspring. While human mothering is a great deal more complex than that of animals, it concerns us that a simple nutritional deficiency can have such a profound effect on instinctive behaviour, particularly since zinc deficiency is considered to be the most widespread deficiency in the Western world. Non-sustainable farming methods, refined foods, cigarettes, alcohol, caffeine, oral contraceptives, inorganic iron supplements, stress, illness and injury are some of the factors that lead to zinc deficiency.

Zinc is also involved in over 200 enzyme functions and is vitally important for every aspect of reproductive health, including breast-feeding. Not surprisingly, pregnant and lactating women have increased requirements for zinc.

Further research shows that the essential mineral manganese, through certain enzymes, also affects the glandular secretions under-lying maternal instinct. Organophosphate pesticides, which are routinely used in non-sustainable agriculture, have been shown to block the uptake of manganese from the soil. So you can see that numerous diet, lifestyle and environmental factors, leading to trace element-deficiencies, can compromise your maternal instinct.

Zinc helps prevent cracked nipples

Adequate zinc levels can help to protect you from cracked nipples. Proper attachment of your newborn to the breast is the best way to avoid this condition (see Chapter 3), but robust nipple tissue is impor-tant too, especially if your baby really likes to suck. His individual temperament will determine how frequently he needs to nurse and you should always remember that babies nurse for comfort as well as nourishment. Some babies seem to be satisfied with brief feeds while others seem to need almost constant oral gratification. (We'll call these higher need babies and we'd have to say that optimally healthy babies often fall into this category.) If your baby is of the latter persuasion, constant nursing at a breast unaccustomed to such things can put a strain on the most robust and zinc-adequate nipple tissue.

Since all our sons were definitely high need, we're glad we knew about the importance of adequate zinc status and we never suffered from cracked nipples.

Adequate zinc for contented babies (and happy mothers)

If you think that new babies are synonymous with crying, we'd like to assure you that this definitely isn't the case. Adequate zinc status can ensure that the two don't go hand in hand. A baby who is zinc-deficient is very jittery and may cry inconsolably. Alone, this crying can give a new mother a good reason for being depressed. If the mother is also zinc-deficient (which is usually why the baby becomes zinc-deficient in the first place) she may be suffering from the baby blues or from the more severe condition, postnatal depression. This duo—a zinc-deficient, depressed mother and a zinc-deficient, endlessly crying baby—are caught in a very vicious cycle indeed. Checking that your own zinc levels are adequate and maintaining those levels can prevent postnatal depression and also ensure that your baby receives sufficient zinc through your breast milk. (For more on treatment of postnatal depression using zinc and other natural remedies see *Healthy Body, Better Birthing.*)

Other benefits of zinc for you and your baby

Because zinc is required for so many aspects of health, you'll find that a baby who has adequate zinc status will be unlikely to suffer from a wide range of so called 'normal' problems. These include skin rashes (such as nappy rash), colic, regurgitation, recurrent infections and oral thrush. Mothers who take zinc supplements not only benefit their babies, but are able to breastfeed for longer periods of time and experience increased energy levels.

Ensuring adequate zinc status

In traditional societies (and in the animal kingdom) zinc deficiency is rarely a problem because the mother usually eats the placenta after giving birth. This organ is the richest source of zinc known—it contains between 350–600 mg of elemental zinc, depending on its size. When the placenta is eaten, adequate zinc status is very quickly restored, maternal zinc stores are established (very important during breastfeeding), and copper levels, which rise during pregnancy, fall back to normal. If you'd like to try this method of re-establishing your zinc status, you can treat the placenta like a piece of liver and fry it with garlic, onions and tomatoes. Alternatively, you can try a stew with mushrooms and red wine (go easy on the alcohol though), or blend it to make a pâté.

Perhaps you can't quite come to grips with the idea of placenta pâté? Relax, there is another option: you can bury the placenta in the garden under a special tree or bush and restore your zinc status through supplementation. Ideally, a zinc supplement should be taken throughout your pregnancy, but if you've already given birth, you can set about restoring your zinc status to adequate levels.

The Zinc Taste Test

To test your zinc status, you can purchase proprietary products from your natural health practitioner, health food store or pharmacy. The products are simple solutions of zinc sulphate heptahydrate (590 mg/100 mL) in purified water. You need to take 5mL of the solution into your mouth and swish it around for one minute.

If you experience a strong, unpleasant taste promptly, your zinc status is adequate, but you'll need to maintain those levels. To do this you can supplement with zinc taken in tablet form. Zinc chelate (along with co-factors such as magnesium, manganese, vitamin B6 and beta-carotene) is the most appropriate supplement and should be taken away from food and other supplements—last thing at night is a good time.

If you experience something more like a dry furry sensation, your zinc status is marginal. If you experience no taste at all then you are zinc-deficient, and in both instances you should supplement using the liquid product (the same one that you just administered for the taste test), as this is more easily absorbed. Alternatively, there are other, more concentrated products that can act quickly to restore zinc status. When you start to experience a strong unpleasant taste promptly, you can revert to supplementing with tablets.

The taste test should be carried out at two-monthly intervals during your pregnancy, although if your pregnancy is well advanced, or if you've already given birth, you might benefit from more frequent testing, and from slightly more aggressive supplementation.

Always make sure that your dose of liquid zinc is well diluted with water (250 mL at least). If you need to take one of the higher dosages of zinc, retest yourself at least once a week and adapt the dosage level appropriately.

THE ZINC TASTE TEST

TEST RESULT	SUPPLEMENT: DOSAGE AND FORM (To be taken separately from food and other supplements)
The taste is strong and prompt (and was also at the last test)	1 zinc tablet daily of 20–25 mg elemental zinc
The taste is strong and prompt (as a result of building zinc status since last test)	2 zinc tablets daily of 20–25 mg elemental zinc
The taste is medium strength with a slightly delayed response	5 mL twice daily
The taste is slight and the response is delayed	10 mL twice daily
There is no taste	20 mL twice daily

NB The liquid measures we give here are only appropriate for the preparation we describe above. Other commercial preparations may be more concentrated and an equivalent, smaller dose can be used.

Interestingly, your level of zinc absorption is nearly twice as high during lactation as it is before conception. The amount of zinc that your baby absorbs from your breast milk is also high (and significantly greater than the absorption from soy or cow's milk formula). However, zinc absorption from breast milk declines over the first 17 weeks of life, as growth rate slows and needs for zinc are reduced.

While it's very important that you ensure that your zinc status is adequate, zinc is just one of many essential nutrients which can contribute to a better breastfeeding experience and a healthier mother and baby. Let's have a look at some of the others.

Nutrients for brain development

Unlike most of your baby's organs, which are fully formed by the end of the first trimester of pregnancy, after which only growth occurs, your baby's brain continues to develop as well as grow throughout the whole of your pregnancy and for the first three years of his life. This development, especially the fine tuning, is dependent on a good supply of the essential fatty acids omega-3 and omega-6. There is considerable uptake of and demand for these nutrients in the last 6 weeks of pregnancy, and if a baby misses out on this phase of development, through premature birth, it is extremely important that these nutrients are delivered in the milk. Breast milk should be rich in these essential fatty acids, but they are usually lacking in infant formulae, although some manufacturers are now aware of the need to ensure their presence. The best supplement to provide you with these nutrients as you approach birth and during the breastfeeding period is one which has a balanced combination of *Evening Primrose* oil and deep-sea fish oils. Make sure to buy a reputable brand of supplement since some fish oils may be contaminated with PCBs, DDT, dioxin or mercury. Zinc, iron and iodine are also important for brain development. As well as testing for zinc status, your midwife or doctor can order a blood test for serum ferritin (iron stores).

Nutrients for hormone production

Just when you think your circulating hormones might return to pre-pregnancy levels, another lot kicks in. Now it's the turn of prolactin, which is the hormone responsible for the production of breast milk, and oxytocin, which is the hormone responsible for the let-down reflex during breastfeeding. This is the same hormone that causes your uterus to contract during labour and also ensures that it returns quickly to its original size. This is one of the reasons why it's important to nurse your baby as soon as possible after the birth.

Because oxytocin is also the hormone that is secreted at orgasm, it's the reason that breastfeeding is such a pleasurable experience. Nature very cleverly designed it that way to ensure the survival of the species, so if you've ever worried about why nursing your baby made you feel so good, relax—it's meant to be like that. It also explains why you might be less interested in your partner while you're breastfeeding. After all you're getting multiple hits of oxytocin every day; again nature ensures that your baby gets all the attention!

Of course these hormones don't materialise out of thin air. Essential fatty acids, vitamins and trace minerals are needed for their production and the hormones for maternal instinct are similarly dependent on adequate levels of various nutrients, as we've already discussed.

Nutrients for energy

All the B-complex vitamins, and minerals such as zinc, magnesium, chromium and manganese are important because they're involved in the metabolism of complex carbohydrates. The complete metabolic break-down of these substances ensures a constant supply of glucose and the energy that your body needs to fuel all of its processes.

ACHIEVING OPTIMUM NUTRITION

If you were diligent about your diet throughout your pregnancy and if you've been taking supplements as our earlier books recommended, then your nutrient levels should be in the optimum range now that you're breastfeeding. If you suffered from morning sickness, or if you've been a bit careless about your food intake, you might have depleted your body's nutrient stores. However, it's never too late for a positive approach. The best way to get all those vital nutrients into your body in a big hurry is through a radical overhaul of your eating habits coupled with comprehensive nutritional supplementation.

Eat fresh, whole and organically grown and fed foods

Try, whenever possible, to select foods which are fresh, in season, unprocessed and organically grown or fed. The reasons are succinctly summed up by the Director of the Institute of Brain Chemistry at Queen Elizabeth Hospital for Children in London, who says that 'Factory farm, intensively produced food is undermining public health and the nation's intelligence.'

Whole, uncontaminated food is high in nutritional value and low in toxins. To help you make positive choices, you can repeat an affirmation such as: 'I am making a positive choice for my health and wellbeing and that of my child' or 'Better diet, better breastfeeding, better baby'.

Avoid allergens

It's important to avoid any foods to which you might be allergic or intolerant while you're breastfeeding. Studies clearly show that this greatly reduces your baby's chances of suffering from atopic eczema. We'll talk more about avoiding allergens in Chapter 10.

Find the correct balance

Just as important as what you should be eating (and what you should be avoiding) is the appropriate balance of all the right foods. When you achieve the appropriate ratio of carbohydrate, protein and fat, you balance two key hormones—insulin and glucagon.

You can think of insulin as the 'saving' hormone; it tells your body to save fat. Glucagon, on the other hand, is the 'spending' hormone; it takes energy from the fat cells to be used as fuel. When these two hormones are well balanced, your blood sugar levels won't fluctuate. Stable blood sugar levels mean you will be less likely to suffer from fatigue and emotional instability. They will ensure that you have plenty of energy to attend to the needs of your new baby (and let's face it, those needs are pretty constant in the early months). They also mean your baby will receive a constant supply of glucose for his energy needs.

Achieving the balance: the Zone Diet

Let's look at the steps involved in achieving that ratio and remember: no more than four hours without a meal or snack!

Protein

First, work out your daily protein requirements. At each meal you need an amount of protein that can fit on, but is no thicker than, the palm of your hand. Now increase that amount by ¼ because you're breastfeeding, by a further ¼ for light activity, by ⅓ for moderate activity (30 minutes of exercise on three days per week) and by ½ for strenuous activity (60 minutes of exercise on five days per week). For a snack, simply halve the amount of protein.

You can use plant (secondary) or animal (primary) protein. Plant proteins are also known as 'incomplete proteins' as they do not contain the full range of essential amino acids, but by combining two of the following food groups over the course of a day you will have a complete protein source, as each group contains a different range of amino acids.

Nuts

These should be raw, unsalted and fresh. Because nuts contain oil, store them in the refrigerator, away from light, and eat them within 2 weeks of purchase. Alternatively, you can buy unshelled nuts and remove the shell as needed. Nuts are a good source of beneficial oils, and you can use them in stir-fries, salads, pasta dishes, and as a snack. (Nuts should never taste bitter as this means the oil has gone rancid.)

Grains and seeds

Whole grains are another source of plant protein (as well as a source of carbohydrate). Eat whole grains such as wholemeal bread, wholemeal pasta and organically grown grains whenever possible in place of white, refined alternatives. (Note that green pasta might not be wholemeal, but white with dye added.) Avoid refined flour products such as cakes, biscuits and pastries because they leach nutrients from your body's stores. Always read bread packets carefully and avoid those that contain preservatives or other additives. Seeds such as pumpkin, sesame, etc, can be used just like nuts—in everything!

Legumes and pulses

Lentils, dried beans, chickpeas, soya, tofu and tempeh are also sources of vegetable protein and have the added benefit of acting as detoxifiers. You should avoid those brands of soy products that might contain genetically engineered beans or high levels of aluminium, fat or sugar. Check labels carefully. The fermented forms of soya (such as tofu or tempeh) are preferred to the original bean, as they don't contain substances called phytates, which can block protein and calcium absorption. If you want to eat the beans, soak them for 24 hours, then throw away the water.

Alternatively, you can eat primary protein. This comes from an animal source, and is a complete protein as it contains all the essential amino acids. Primary proteins are contained in the following foods.

Fish
Eat fish at least 2–3 times weekly. Fish is low in saturated fats and high in essential fatty acids. Especially beneficial are the deep-sea, ocean and cold-water fish (e.g. mackerel, mullet, salmon, tailor, trevally and sardines) which are also less polluted than other types. You should avoid large fish (e.g. tuna and swordfish) which may contain high levels of mercury. Fresh fish are definitely preferable to tinned or frozen fish.

Chicken
Eat free-range and organically fed poultry only. The two are not necessarily the same thing, as some free-range poultry are fed hormones and antibiotics. Trim off the skin to avoid unhealthy fats.

Eggs
Eggs are an excellent source of protein. Limit their consumption only if they cause gastro-intestinal problems such as constipation or gas. Make sure eggs come from poultry that are free-range and organically fed.

Dairy foods
Avoid cow's milk and cheese. Goat's (or soya) milk and cheese are preferable. Cow's milk products can create excessive mucus and are also a factor in many malabsorption problems. They can also adversely affect your breastfeeding baby. Natural cultured acidophilus or bifidus non-flavoured yoghurt is a good choice.

Red meat
Eat red meat in moderation. Lean meat with the fat trimmed, and game meats, are best. Unless you are certain that the animal from which meat is taken has been organically fed, avoid organ meats, sausage and mince. Organ meats contain high levels of pesticides and hormones. Some butchers make their own gourmet sausages (which contain good quantities of meat, although they are still high in fat and may contain offal) and if you want mince, you can ask your butcher to mince a selected lean (non-offal) cut on site. You should avoid delicatessen meats, which are high in fats, organ meats and toxic preservatives.

Carbohydrates

Once you've selected your protein portion, the next step is to add your carbohydrates. Carbohydrate foods include vegetables, grains and sugars. Vegetables are the preferred form in a healthy diet, with whole grains making up the balance. But even within these preferred forms, there are two types of carbohydrates: risk-reducing (low glycaemic) or risk-promoting (high glycaemic). The category into which a particular food falls depends on the amount of carbohydrate present in the food and the amount of fibre it contains. (See Appendix 4 for details.) Low carbohydrate foods with high fibre and water contents are risk-reducing and it is these foods which you should select whenever possible. Risk-reducing vegetables include asparagus, bok choy, broccoli, brussel sprouts, cabbage, capsicum, cauliflower, cucumber, eggplant, lettuce, mushrooms, onion, spinach and tomatoes.

You should eat lots of vegetables from this category every day. Select a wide variety, especially those that are dark green and leafy or red or orange, as well as avocado, which is also a good source of essential fatty acids. Pale lettuce is not highly nutritious. Eat both raw and cooked vegetables on a regular basis. You can add chopped fresh herbs (e.g. parsley and watercress) for interest and flavour.

You might like to try vegetable juices as a great way of ensuring adequate vegetable intake. Carrot, celery and beetroot taste good, but any vegetable you have in your fridge can be added.

Risk-reducing fruits include apples, apricots, berries, grapes, some melons, oranges, peaches, pineapple and strawberries. You should eat no more than 2–3 pieces of fruit daily as fruit is high in sugar (and provides no nutrients that aren't also available from vegetables). This includes fruit that is juiced, which should be diluted 50:50 with purified water. Avoid dried fruit, which is high in sugar and usually contains preservatives (or else is mouldy).

Moderate risk foods (which can still be eaten, but in smaller amounts) include baked beans, corn, carrots, peas, potatoes, squash, sweet potato, bananas, dates, figs, mango, papaya, fruit juices and wholegrain pastas, breads and cereal grains (wholegrain of course).

Refined carbohydrates such as sugars, white bread, refined pastas and white rice strip important nutrients from your body and should be avoided. Bear in mind that most Australian diets are too high in carbo-hydrates and too low in protein. If you aim for a ratio of 1:1 you will probably get the balance approximately right.

Healthy fats

Once you've selected your protein and carbohydrates you need to add healthy fats to each meal since the walls of every cell in your body contain a lipid (fat) layer and fats are also necessary to tell your brain that you have had enough to eat. They reduce your blood sugar and insulin response to a meal and are a very important part of achieving the balance between insulin and glucagon. Remember, they're important for your baby's brain and eye development too. Here is a list of healthy fats and oils.

- For dressings use olive, flax, pumpkin, walnut, safflower and sunflower oils (all cold-pressed). These are high in essential fatty acids if not heated. Keep them in the fridge (except olive oil) in dark containers. Add lemon, pepper, garlic and herbs to taste.

- For cooking use olive and sesame oils (these do not saturate on heating).

- Choose flax, pumpkin, sesame and sunflower seeds.

- Choose walnuts, hazelnuts and almonds.

- Avocado is a source of healthy fat.

- Eggless or soya mayonnaise is a good choice.

Snacks

You can have snacks in between meals. You shouldn't go more than 4 hours without food. For a snack, work out the appropriate proportions in the same way, but halve your protein allowance.

Water

Finally, you need to drink plenty of purified water. Drink 8–12 glasses (2–3 litres) every day. Spring water is a reasonable substitute. Mineral water is okay occasionally, but may be high in salt. Unpurified tap water is high in many toxins and heavy metals that become concentrated, not destroyed, by boiling. Make sure that you drink between meals so that the water doesn't interfere with your digestion. On hot days, increase your intake so that your breast milk is suitably dilute for your baby who will be thirstier than usual due to the heat. Remember, it's important to drink lots of water to produce plenty of breast milk; it is *not* necessary to drink milk to produce breast milk.

This method of eating (and drinking) is known as the Zone Insulin System or the Zone Diet and you'll certainly have a better breastfeeding experience if you always stay in the Zone.

As well as telling you what to eat, we should also mention what to avoid, though you'll probably know already that most foods on this list are not good for you.

Foods to avoid

⚶ Avoid saturated fats. These will upset your prostaglandin–hormone–mineral balance. This means avoiding heated and animal fats.

⚶ Avoid eating fried food, except stir-fries. Cook with olive oil, which is a mono-unsaturated oil and will not saturate on heating. Sesame oil is an alternative.

⚶ Avoid butter and margarine. They are both saturated fats. Margarine is worse than butter as not only does it saturate during processing but it is also full of chemicals. Try avocado, banana, hummus, tahini or nut spreads instead. Nut spreads must be fresh, refrigerated and kept away from light.

⚶ Avoid sugar and all sweet things, including honey, sugar substitutes, undiluted fruit juices, cakes, biscuits, pastries and soft drinks. Sugar leaches essential nutrients from your body, and increases your insulin response. Read labels carefully. Sugar has lots of other names, e.g. dextrose, glucose, fructose (and other words ending in 'ose'), cornstarch, malt, molasses etc.

⚶ Only add salt to taste. Do not use it routinely in cooking or on food. Use rock, sea or Celtic salt rather than ordinary table salt. Avoid highly salted, pre-prepared food.

⚶ Avoid junk foods; they usually fall into high saturated fat, high salt, high sugar, low nutrient categories. Read labels carefully and avoid additives.

⚶ Avoid caffeine and alcohol. We'll talk about the reasons for completely avoiding these two drugs in Chapter 6.

How to prepare your food

If you buy your fresh food from a shop with a high turnover and you eat it as soon as possible, it will be more nutritious. You need both raw and cooked foods, but overcooking can destroy nutrients. Lots of foods can be eaten raw, including all vegetables except potatoes. However root vegetables, such as carrots, need to be broken down in some way such as lightly cooking (steaming or stir-frying), grating or juicing them in order for you to be able to digest them properly. If you microwave your food, even to defrost or heat it, you destroy the protein and there's also the possibility of exposure to harmful radiation.

Take your supplements

Breastfeeding puts increased demands on your nutritional stores, which have just been depleted by pregnancy and birth. In fact, the demand for nutrients is even greater when you are breastfeeding than it was while you were pregnant. While the best way to get all those nutrients is from the sort of diet we've just outlined, supplements are important to make up for any shortfall. Ideally, supplementation should continue throughout the whole period of breastfeeding, and we'd actually suggest forever! The table below sets out the dosages of supplements appropriate for a breastfeeding mother. There are numerous proprietary preparations that contain combinations of these ingredients. Ask your health practitioner for guidance and take as directed.

SUPPLEMENTS FOR BREASTFEEDING MOTHERS

SUPPLEMENT	DAILY DOSAGE
Vitamin A	10 000 IU, or 6 mg beta-carotene (choose mixed carotenes if available)
Vitamin B complex	B1, B2, B3, B6: 50 mg each
	B5: 100 mcg
	B12: 400 mcg
	Biotin: 100 mcg
	Choline, inositol, PABA: 50 mg
	Folic acid: 500 mcg
Vitamin C	1000–2000 mg (1–2 g). Take the higher dose temporarily if you are suffering from infection.

Bioflavonoids	400–1000 mg
Vitamin D	200 IU
Vitamin E	600 IU
Vitamin K	2.5 mcg
Calcium	800 mg
Magnesium	400 mg (half the dose of calcium)
Potassium	50 mg or as cell salt (potassium chloride, 3 tablets)
Iron	Supplement only if need is proven; dosage depends on serum ferritin levels (stored iron) and should be chelated (organic). If levels < 30 mcg per litre, take 30 mg If levels < 45 mcg per litre, take 20 mg If levels < 60 mcg per litre, take 10 mg
Manganese	25 mg
Zinc	25–60 mg. Take on an empty stomach, and separately from food and other supplements. Dose level to depend on result of Zinc Taste Test. See earlier in this chapter.
Chromium	100–400 mcg. The upper limit is for those with sugar cravings or with proven need.
Selenium	100–200 mcg. The upper limit is for those exposed to high levels of heavy metal or chemical pollution. Seleno-methionine is the most stable and useful form of this mineral. Sodium selemite is less useful and must be taken separately from vitamin C and zinc.
Iodine	10 mcg or take 150 mg of kelp instead
Acidophilus / Bifidus (lactobacilli)	Half to one teaspoonful of each, one to three times daily. The upper limits are for those who suffer from thrush.
Evening primrose oil/ flaxseed oil	400 mg two to three times daily
EPA/DHA (deep sea fish oils)	600 mg two to three times daily, especially if your diet contains little deep-sea fish.
Garlic	2000–5000 mg. The higher levels are for those exposed to toxins.
Silica	20 mg

Copper	1–2 mg, but only if zinc levels are adequate
Hydrochloric acid and	
digestive enzymes	For those with digestive problems—take according to directions on the label

Vitamins A and E are fat soluble and are therefore transferred efficiently through the breast milk so don't exceed our recommended dosages. If you're using vitamin E on your nipples, make sure it's washed off before nursing. Vitamin D is secreted into the breast milk in limited concentrations, and is safe at the recommended dosage. However, excessive dosages can lead to elevated calcium in the infant and should be avoided. Most other vitamins and minerals are released in controlled amounts into the breast milk and there is no possibility of an overdose.

Vitamin B6 is required in greater amounts during lactation and is therefore an important supplement at this time, but in very high doses (500 mg or more) it can suppress prolactin and therefore affect milk production. Keep to the dosage that we recommend. Vitamin B12 deficiency is very dangerous to an infant, and vegetarian mothers have an even greater need than others to supplement with this nutrient.

Finally, remember to check your zinc and stored iron (ferritin) levels regularly throughout the breastfeeding period and supplement accordingly.

IF YOUR BABY HAS A TUMMY UPSET

If your baby has strong immune and gastrointestinal systems (he will if you had good preconception and pregnancy care), he will probably cope well with whatever you eat. But some foods such as spices, raw onions and vegetables from the brassica family (cabbage, cauliflower, broccoli and brussel sprouts) are problematic for many babies, and you may need to restrict these in your diet. If your baby has a problem—diarrhoea or an upset stomach—look first at what you've been eating. It may not be what you ate that day as the effect can be delayed by 2–3 days.

Eating well and taking your supplements is important for an adequate supply of nutritious breast milk, but you need to consider how your lifestyle can affect the quality of your milk and the success of your breastfeeding relationship.

A healthy lifestyle for better breastfeeding

If you're reading this book before you've even conceived (don't laugh, Jan read *Raising your Talented Child* long before she was pregnant) then you've got the perfect opportunity to practise preconception health care which is the very best foundation for a better breastfeeding experience. It's often much simpler to implement the appropriate changes, which include an improved diet, a healthier lifestyle and a cleaner environment, in those months before you conceive. These measures can also be more effective if implemented fully then, because they can involve both you and your partner equally. You'll be in the quest for a 'better' pregnancy, birth, bonding and breastfeeding relationship together. So if you're not pregnant now, give yourself a minimum period of four months before you make any attempt to conceive. Start to eat—and live—healthily now, and ideally you'll follow the same healthy diet and lifestyle throughout your pregnancy and beyond. For all the details of what to do and how to do it, you should read our earlier books *Healthy Parents, Better Babies, Healthy Lifestyle, Better Pregnancy*, and *Healthy Body, Better Birthing*.

But if you're already pregnant, or if you're dealing with a

breastfeeding relationship that isn't going quite the way you'd hoped, or if you're doing just fine but want to make sure that you can continue for as long as you can, we'll give you the rundown on all the dos and don'ts of a healthy lifestyle which will help you establish and maintain a successful breastfeeding relationship.

SUBSTANCES TO AVOID WHEN YOU'RE BREASTFEEDING

It's probably stating the obvious, but when you're breastfeeding it's important that you avoid all of the things that (we hope) you avoided when you were pregnant. That includes cigarettes, alcohol, caffeine and other drugs. Just because you can hold your baby in your arms doesn't mean that he's been removed from the ill effects of these unhealthy lifestyle factors. Not only do they have an adverse effect on your breastfeeding baby, they can also seriously compromise your nutritional status. Even an occasional lapse on your part (or your partner's) may well affect your baby adversely, even up to a couple of days after you slip up.

Alcohol

Alcohol is a depressant and is transmitted through the breast milk to your baby, making him drowsy and unable to feed properly. It is toxic to his brain and his liver, can lead to psychomotor problems and it leaches nutrients from your body as well as his, as it is a refined carbohydrate. It may also reduce your milk supply and affect your let-down mechanism. Quite apart from the effects of alcohol on your breast milk, recent research suggests that the mere smell of alcohol may prime infants to become heavy drinkers as adults. Most commercial alcohol drinks also contain additives and potentially harmful chemicals. It takes two hours for your body to break down one standard drink, during which time the transfer to your milk will be high.

Caffeine

Caffeine is a stimulant and will make your baby very jumpy and irritable. It also increases the excretion of nutrients from your body.

However, if you simply must drink tea (not coffee), two cups of weak tea daily (not more) are acceptable. Choose a tea that is naturally low in caffeine (not decaffeinated) and preferably organically grown and contained in unbleached bags. Green and herb teas are preferable; see Chapter 4 for some suggestions about herb teas that will help with milk production.

We don't recommend decaffeinated tea or coffee because of the chemicals used to remove the caffeine. Even if decaffeinated through a natural, water-based process, the tea or coffee will contain other harmful constituents, which become more active during this procedure. Cereal-based substitutes and *Dandelion Root* coffee are fine, but check that they do not contain added sugar. Remember, caffeine is a constituent of many soft drinks, which of course you should avoid anyway because of the sugar content.

Smoking

Smoking is banned; that applies to your partner too. Nicotine is a drug that can affect your baby in the same way it affects you—adversely! It can lead to vomiting, diarrhoea, rapid heartbeat and restlessness in the infant if transmitted through the breast milk. We won't bother to tell you about the effects of the 4000 odd other chemicals contained in cigarette smoke. But amongst the many infant problems associated with maternal (and paternal) smoking are bronchitis, asthma, pneumonia, SIDS and higher risks of lung cancer in later life. Smoking can also affect your milk production. Passive smoking is also a problem (which is why your partner shouldn't smoke), so make sure you and your baby avoid smoky environments.

Recreational drugs

All recreational drugs are on the prohibited list. This means not only hard drugs like heroin, but also soft drugs such as marijuana, which is transmitted through your milk to your baby, causing sleepiness and weakness and affecting his ability to feed. It may also affect your milk production through its inhibiting action on prolactin. Marijuana stays in your body for a least a month as it is absorbed into fatty tissue. Hard drugs, of course, are extremely dangerous and can cause addiction in a breastfeeding infant.

Oral contraceptives

Oral contraceptives, even the low-dose mini-pill, should be avoided. One of the main threats to the nutritional content of your breast milk is the use of the mini-pill, commonly prescribed during breastfeeding. We'll discuss this further in Chapter 9, along with the effect of synthetic hormones on your baby. Luckily, there are natural alternative methods of contraception (see Chapter 9 for more on this, too). However, if you're fully breastfeeding, your need for any form of contraception is substantially reduced, and it will be a lot easier for you to avoid this chemical threat to your baby's (and your) health.

Prescribed medication

If you have to take a course of prescribed medication, always remember to tell your doctor that you're breastfeeding, and that you want to continue. The need to take prescribed medication is no reason to stop nursing, but the drug choice will need to be made thoughtfully, length of use carefully monitored and your baby closely observed. We've included a list of commonly prescribed pharmaceuticals and their suitability for use during breastfeeding in Appendix 1.

Herbal remedies

Many herbal constituents are excreted in breast milk and are thus transmitted from mother to baby while nursing, though usually in very reduced amounts. While this can usefully constitute a method for treating the baby (by having the mother ingest the remedy), it also means you need to take care. Just because a medicinal remedy or supplement is natural, doesn't necessarily mean it's non-toxic. There are remedies of herbal origin which have been shown by traditional use or scientific testing to be safe (these are the ones we suggest for use throughout the book) and there are others which, by the same means, are contraindicated during breastfeeding or that need to be used with caution. It's often just a matter of dosage. We've included a list of potentially unsafe herbal substances in Appendix 2. We've also included a list of commonly used herbs (for general health conditions) which are safe to take. For any others, consult a naturopath or herbalist.

Note that culinary use of herbs is usually safe, but avoid *Sage* as it dries up your milk. Remember, too, that herbal teas must be checked for suitability.

Any individual can have an allergic reaction to a plant, so exclude from your diet any plants to which you know you are allergic. If your baby shows distress after using any remedy, herbal or otherwise, discontinue its use and seek professional advice.

CAN I BREASTFEED WITH A DISEASE OR INFECTION?

There are some diseases and infections that can be transmitted through the breast milk, and others which can't. In some instances, HIV for example, there is controversy and different studies give different information. We've listed in Appendix 3 some conditions which may concern you—but this list does not replace the advice of a medical practitioner. Remember that breastfeeding confers considerable immune protection upon your baby, and this needs to be a part of any decision you make as to whether you breastfeed or not.

STRIVE FOR A CLEAN ENVIRONMENT FREE OF TOXINS

As the preconception, pregnancy and breastfeeding months and years together define the beginning and end of the most critical time of growth in the human life cycle, it's only sensible that you and your baby stay as free of toxins as possible during these times. You were probably careful to avoid environmental pollution when you were pregnant (and, we hope, before you conceived), so don't stop now. If you didn't take care before, all the more reason to start now.

It's vital to eat a healthy diet and avoid drugs as we've already explained, but that's not the whole story. Our world is becoming more and more toxic and full of potentially harmful substances. These are often difficult to avoid, as they come through the food we eat, the water we drink and the air we breathe. Unfortunately, breast milk, because it contains fat, can act as a storehouse for toxins. Your fatty tissue is also a reservoir for these substances, and as it breaks down to aid in the production of breast milk it can release the toxins that have accumulated over a period of time. More than 350 man-made chemicals and pollutants have been found in breast milk, including pesticides, perfumes, disinfectants, suntan oils and industrial raw materials.

This sounds alarming, but there is some good news. Studies which have compared children fed breast milk with those fed formula have found that even when the breast milk contains higher levels of toxins than the formula, the children are still better off as far as health, behaviour and wellbeing are concerned. This is assumed to be due to the protective, nutritional and other benefits of breast milk. Furthermore, only between 1 and 10 per cent of most substances taken in by the mother will find their way through the breast membrane into the milk, so the levels of toxins reaching your baby are much lower than those reaching you. You can rest assured that breastfeeding remains far and away the best way to feed and nourish your baby, but you must do all you can to protect the quality of your breast milk.

Children are more vulnerable to toxins than adults, not only because they are still forming vital body organs and systems but because they have faster metabolisms and less well developed immune systems. A healthy baby can deal with a 'reasonable' load of toxins, but problems and developmental disorders can be triggered by an overload. Environmental toxins can contribute to the development of these conditions in babies and children:

- Sudden Infant Death Syndrome (SIDS)
- developmental and sensory problems
- sleep problems, hyperactivity
- poor co-ordination
- poor organ and system function

Environmental toxins may also lead to your baby having a greater risk of developing these conditions in later life:

- aggression, emotional and social problems
- Attention Deficit Disorder
- learning and speech problems, dyslexia, reduced IQ
- immune dysfunction, allergy, asthma
- reproductive and sexual problems
- cancer in childhood, later life or the next generation

- autism, schizophrenia, depression
- chronic fatigue syndrome, chemical sensitivity
- hypertension

So you can see how important it is to put in place as much protection as possible. However, despite your desire to give your baby the cleanest possible breast milk, now, unfortunately, is not the time to detoxify. Breast milk is a major channel for toxic waste, as we have seen, so a detoxification program will make the problem worse. Prevention is the best approach, along with the use of antioxidants: nutrients such as vitamins A, C and E and zinc and selenium. Other useful measures include taking gentle liver herbs such as *Dandelion Root* tea, drinking lots of purified water, exercising and making sure you have regular bowel motions to clear your digestive tract.

How can you prevent exposure to toxins? Let's look first at the main toxins, and how you are exposed through your food, through your drinking water, in your home and during recreation. Then we'll try and give you some ideas about how to protect yourself and your baby from their ill effects.

WHAT ARE THE ENVIRONMENTAL TOXINS I MUST AVOID?

Heavy metals

Heavy metals are those which are toxic to humans, and for which your body has no metabolic pathway. They can be found in all body systems, and are not eliminated by any normal physiological process. They can be removed through various detoxification measures, but as detox is not appropriate during breastfeeding, avoidance is what you need to focus on. Also keep taking your antioxidants and follow our other recommendations below.

Lead

As lead is one of the most problematic metals, we'll look at it in some detail. Much of what we say about lead also applies to the other heavy metals. Lead is found in the following substances and situations:

- paint (of pre-1970 manufacture)
- pesticides and fertilisers (which means you can ingest traces of lead through your food if it's not organic)
- food tins (especially if they are damaged as lead lines the seams, and acidic foods will leach the lead out into the food)
- pottery and china (especially if old, highly glossy and multicoloured as lead used to be used, and sometimes still is, in coloured glazes)
- some toiletries (some mascaras, hair colours)
- some hobby and craft materials (e.g. leadlighting)
- batteries (car and industrial)
- drinking water (as lead solder is used on water pipes and fluoridation increases lead absorption)
- traffic exhaust (from leaded petrol)
- bone meal (sometimes used for calcium and magnesium supplements)
- smoke (from cigarettes and coal burning)
- lead crystal (often used in glassware)

Lead transfers to breast milk in the same proportion as it occurs in maternal blood, and children absorb 50 per cent of the lead entering their bodies compared with the 10 per cent absorbed by adults. It then stores in various tissues, accumulating in the brain, peripheral nervous system, bones and bone marrow, gastrointestinal tract and kidneys. The principal storage site is the skeleton. Most of the problems that we've already discussed can be the result of lead toxicity. These include central nervous system and brain damage; learning difficulties, mental difficulties, reduced intelligence and hyperactivity; behavioural problems, aggression, destructive behaviour, temper tantrums and irritability; insomnia and drowsiness; poor motor co-ordination and lack of sensory perception; loss of appetite, constipation and diarrhoea; anaemia; liver and kidney dysfunction; increased allergy and frequent infections; recurrent fits; cancer and dental decay. In later life, lead toxicity can predispose a person to cardiovascular problems, hypertension, depression, anxiety, poor concentration and memory problems.

What you can do to minimise lead toxicity
In order to avoid these problems, you'll need to avoid contact with the substances we've listed above. One of the most important things to avoid is sanding or stripping back lead-based paint. You should also

keep your car windows shut when you're in heavy traffic, and if you live near a busy road and need to open your windows, frequently use a wet mop on floors and a damp cloth on surfaces to keep them free of lead residues, and place net curtains on your windows to catch the dust. Purify all your water (we'll talk more about this in a while), and don't grow your own vegetables if you live near a major road.

Nutrients that reduce lead absorption include calcium, magnesium, phosphorus, iron, zinc and copper. All the antioxidants, especially selenium, zinc and vitamins C and E, help to protect you from the ill effects of lead, as do the B-complex vitamins and chromium. Pectin, (found in apples stewed with their pips) bananas, onions and garlic are helpful foods, and it's important to have a diet that's not too low (or too high) in protein. The levels we suggest in Chapter 5 are just right. You should also avoid a high level of fats which act as a reservoir for toxins of all kinds. Heavy metals are dissolved more easily in acidic conditions. In order to avoid this problem it's important to eat the way we suggest (which will avoid your system becoming too acidic) and purify your water (in case your water supply contains acids).

Mercury

The main sources of mercury contamination are:

- dental fillings (amalgam contains mercury)
- large fish (such as tuna, swordfish and shark, which are at the top of the feeding chain)
- bottom-dwelling fish (including crustaceans)
- the electronic industry (also batteries in electronic games)
- some paints
- fluorescent lights
- some pesticides, insecticides and fungicides
- the water supply (because of run-off from agriculture)
- some medications and spermicides
- photographic and printing processes

By far the most common source of contamination is dental fillings. But now is not a good time to have those fillings replaced or drilled as mercury vapour will be released. You should also avoid chewing on gum, which increases the vapour release from amalgam six-fold. If you need dental work go to a dentist who works with amalgam removal and explain your situation. He or she will have equipment that helps to limit the problem.

Mercury accumulates in the kidneys, liver and brain (especially the pituitary gland). One German study found that concentrations in these organs in deceased foetuses, newborns and young children were in direct proportion to the number of amalgam fillings in the mothers' mouths. Problems associated with mercury poisoning include behavioural problems, nervous system problems, problems with movement control, problems with speech, language, attention and memory, psychological, emotional and mood disorders, spinal and motor neurone disease, auto-immune disease, kidney disease, multiple sclerosis, cardiovascular disease, hypertension, impairment of hearing and colour perception, congenitally damaged teeth and serious degenerative diseases.

What you can do to minimise mercury toxicity
If you have a lot of fillings, don't despair. Levels of vulnerability vary from person to person. However, it's very important to keep your zinc status adequate, and take plenty of vitamin C and selenium. A garlic supplement may also be helpful. Good foods to eat to protect against mercury toxicity include eggs, legumes, onions, asparagus, brussel sprouts and cabbage.

Aluminium
The main sources of aluminium contamination are:

- cookware (saucepans, teapots and aluminium foil, especially if acid foods are cooked in them)
- antiperspirants (especially sprays, which you can inhale)
- food additives (colours and preservatives)
- antacids and toothpastes
- processed cheese
- some medicines (especially those for diarrhoea)
- some soya milks
- tetra packs which contain acidic fruit juices
- powders such as milk powders, white flour and baking powder which need to run freely (aluminium absorbs moisture)
- drinking water (aluminium is used as an anti-frothing and foaming agent)

Aluminium accumulates in the brain, parathyroid, bones, lungs, muscles, liver, kidneys and colon, and leads to various ill effects including mineral loss from bones, gastrointestinal disturbances, skin problems, fatigue, encephalopathy, kidney problems and lung disease.

What you can do to minimise aluminium toxicity
To help protect your body and your breast milk from aluminium, take plenty of vitamin C, zinc, selenium, magnesium, manganese, calcium and vitamin D. Silica is a mineral which seems to protect against aluminium absorption and can be obtained from health food shops as a tissue salt.

Cadmium
The main source of cadmium toxicity is cigarette smoking (both active and passive). We feel we've warned you against that enough already! Other sources include:

- drinking water (as cadmium is contained in some plumbing alloys)
- some paints, batteries, electronic equipment, TV sets
- photographic processing chemicals
- electroplating, rustproofing, welding, solders
- fungicides, pesticides
- some ceramics
- shredded rubber tyres and dust near highways
- some tools (which are coated with cadmium)

Cadmium accumulates in the liver and kidneys and has been shown to affect emotional, nervous system and mental development.

What you can do to minimise cadmium toxicity
Take plenty of chromium, zinc, calcium and vitamin C, and adequate (but not excessive) levels of copper and iron. Good foods to combat cadmium include eggs, onions and garlic.

Copper
Copper isn't really a heavy metal, but in excess it causes zinc deficiency, amongst other problems. It's an important nutrient at moderate

levels of ingestion, but is often found in high concentrations due to its vast number of sources which include:

* the oral contraceptive pill (which does not actually contain copper, but causes levels in the body to rise)
* copper intra-uterine contraceptive devices (IUDs)
* the water supply (copper piping is common)
* copper cookware
* copper jewellery
* hair dyes containing henna
* swimming pools (which use a copper salt as an algaecide)

Some of the ill effects of high copper levels include thyroid dysfunction, postnatal depression, anaemia, dermatitis and allergies.

What you can do to minimise copper toxicity
To protect yourself and your baby from the ill effects of excess copper, take plenty of zinc and continue to assess your zinc status. Other important nutrients to combat copper include vitamin C, manganese, selenium, calcium, molybdenum and vitamin B5.

Testing for heavy metal exposure
Heavy metals can be assessed through blood tests and hair analysis. Blood tests will only show the level of metals present on the day of testing, whereas hair analysis will assess more accurately the load in the body's tissues. Now may not be the best time to find out if you have a high load, since you can't undergo detoxification without stopping feeding. However, in cases of extreme toxicity, this could be considered. You'd then need to express your milk (see Chapter 4) to keep the production up and resume breastfeeding after detoxification was complete. (Of course you would have to dispose of the tainted expressed milk.) This would mean that you'd need to choose a very fast method for detoxification such as chelation. This is a process whereby an agent is introduced into your body, through an oral or intravenous pathway, to bind to the metal and remove it. Unless you really need to undertake such drastic action, the best course is to keep taking your antioxidant nutrient supplements, and follow our other recommendations.

Pesticides

According to the World Health Organisation, pesticide residues are the most common of all chemicals found in breast milk. (In the category of pesticides we include non-organic fertilisers and other agro-chemicals as well as insecticides, fungicides and herbicides.) In fact the levels of DDT and dieldrin and some other pesticides in breast milk have been found to be up to twice those in the mother's blood.

If you spray the plants in your garden, if you use pest control in your home, if you spray or bomb to kill flying insects, fleas or cockroaches, if you treat your pets with washes or flea collars, if you eat non-organic foods, if you live in the country near any area which is sprayed or if you are a farmer spraying crops or treating livestock, then you come into contact with considerable levels of pesticides. Even if you do none of these things, if you don't purify your water, you'll get zapped, as pesticide residue is present in rain water, is not filtered from public water supplies, and drains off agricultural areas which surround rivers and reservoirs. Some crops are sprayed up to 15 times when in the ground and then are sprayed again when they are stored.

Pesticides are neurotoxic and affect the developing brain and nervous system, and some of the adverse effects include neuro-developmental impairment, learning problems, physical co-ordination problems, immune dysfunction and permanent loss of brain function if there is a high level of contamination during pregnancy and the first three years of life.

Organophosphates, which work by inactivating enzyme systems in pests, have been implicated in the inactivation of enzyme systems in humans, in central nervous system damage, mental problems, damage to eyes, bladder, heart, autonomic ganglia and skeletal muscle, in muscular dystrophy, multiple sclerosis and problems in the respiratory, cardiovascular, skeletal and immune systems. Lindane has been associated with cancer, and kepane and DBCP with testicular damage.

What you can do to avoid pesticide toxicity

To avoid these dangerous chemicals, eat organic foods and peel vegetables and fruits or wash them with a solution of vinegar and purified water. Also use the alternative forms of pest control listed below. Some essential oils and herbs can prevent insects from invading your home—and they smell good too!

Personal repellents
- *Stinking Roger*, but this has an unpleasant smell, so you may prefer to choose one of the others
- *Citronella*
- *Pennyroyal*
- *Huon Pine* oil
- *Lavender* oil

Don't rub these directly on to your baby, but use them nearby, and add some lavender to the last rinse when you wash his clothes.

To repel mosquitoes
- *Paperbark* oil
- *Mimosa* flowers
- *Balm of Gilead*
- *Pennyroyal* leaves (fresh or dried)
- *Lavender*

To repel flies
- *Eucalyptus* oil

- *Citronella*
- *Tansy* (but this can irritate skin)
- *Basil*
- *Pennyroyal* oil
- *Bergamot* oil
- *Horehound*
- *Cloves*
- *Stinking Roger*

To repel moths
- *Garlic*
- *Bay* leaves
- *Sassafras* leaves

To repel ants
- *Red Pepper*
- *camphor*
- *borax*
- ground *Cloves*

To repel silverfish
- *Lavender* oil
- *Bay* leaves

Use fly swats to deal with flying insects, and block openings that cockroaches and ants use to enter your home. Lights with a reddish rather than blue tinge will attract fewer flying insects. If you have a persistent infestation, find one of the pest control companies that use ecological pest control, but be very careful what you agree to. For example, pyrethrum, a natural pesticide derived from plants, is toxic to humans as well as insects (though less so than chemical insecticides). Ask the pest controllers to use a gas rather than a spray so there's no residue, and move out while the work is being done. (An advantage of using a gas is that you won't need to cover all your kitchen equipment.) Before you return home, get someone to open up all the windows and doors for several hours. Then use some of the natural repellents we've suggested to keep the insects away. Be aware that fumes from chemical pesticides sprayed under your house can penetrate the floor and permeate your living spaces.

Hormone disruptors

In the first few months of your baby's development, all his hormone receptor sites are forming, so this is not a good time for exposure to chemicals or other substances which can mimic hormones or disrupt the development process. Even slight exposure to disruptors can trigger a hormonal response which can lead to a cascade of effects. Disruptors can also affect brain growth.

What are hormone disruptors? Heavy metals, pesticides, solvents, chemicals such as PCBs and phthalates found in plastics, styrenes which are found in foam-based materials and some industrial pollutants are amongst the offenders. Then there are hormones themselves, which can be found in foods from an animal source, the water supply (as it is contaminated by run-off containing animal and human urine) and hormonal medications such as the contraceptive pill.

Hormone-like substances can also be found in plants. They are quite weak in their effects, but we discuss our concerns about feeding your baby substantial amounts of soya foods in Chapter 8.

What you can do to avoid hormone disruptors

Purify your water, avoid plastic containers for your food, replace foam-based furniture and avoid the solvents, heavy metals and pesticides we've warned you about already and you will have removed a large part of the problem.

Other dangerous chemicals

We are exposed to a chemical cocktail every day of our lives. Because of synergistic effects, contact with quite small amounts of even two chemicals simultaneously can magnify the danger to us to more than a thousand times that of exposure to the single substances. Most scientific laboratory studies for toxicity only test chemicals singly, which is not the way we encounter them in our daily lives. The following list highlights dangerous chemicals which you may encounter in isolation, but will more usually come across in combination with other dangerous substances. Either way, they are to be avoided if possible.

- Solvents cross over into the breast milk at three times the level found in the mother's blood.
- Plasticisers, added to plastics for flexibility, are used for food containers and contaminate the food.
- Dioxins which are produced when plastics are burned (such as in public incinerators) are found in high levels in breast milk and can cause cancer and retard intellectual development.
- PCBs (polychlorinated biphenyls), used in many plastics, have been shown to interfere with dental development, neurological development and cognitive function, causing learning problems and reduced IQ, and can cross over into the breast milk at levels four to ten times higher than that in the mother's blood.
- Vinyl chloride, used in more than half of all plastic products, has been linked to many developmental problems. (Polyvinylchloride has not.)
- Solvents such as benzene and toluene have been linked with cancer, among other problems.
- Formaldehyde, found in many domestic products, causes nausea, headaches, dizziness, breathing difficulties and depression, can lead to chemical sensitivity and is a suspected carcinogen.

Many of these chemicals can be found in your home, as we shall see.

Contamination through your food

Toxic residues in foods include pesticides, herbicides, antibiotics, hormones and additives. Foods are tested for unacceptable levels of these substances, but the standard used is set for adults, so where the transfer rate into your milk is high, your baby will receive far more than the proportional amount. That's assuming that there is a safe level of any of these pollutants, which is, of course, debatable.

Making sure your food is safe

Buy organic foods

By simply shopping at an organic supplier, you can reduce your exposure to pesticides, herbicides, antibiotics, hormones and additives. Since fat is the reservoir for most toxins, it's extremely important that the foods you buy that are from an animal source are organic. If you can't buy organic meat, for example, restrict your animal foods and trim all fats. Be aware that there are many misleading names for foods that make them sound organic, such as 'free-range' (this refers to where the animal is kept, not what it's fed), and 'vegetarian' or 'grain-fed' (which doesn't exclude hormones and antibiotics). You need to check that your food is certified as organic.

Read labels carefully

The debate about genetically engineered foods continues, with regard to environmental hazards as well as health concerns. However, since we have, as yet, little idea about how these foods may affect us or our children (through breast milk), we strongly suggest that you do your best to avoid them. Because of concerns regarding cross-contamination you cannot be confident of avoiding these foods however diligent you are at reading labels. We suggest shopping at health food and organic stores where you can be confident of the purity of the products, and choosing those that are certified as free from genetically modified ingredients.

Many food additives such as preservatives, colouring, flavourings, emulsifiers, extenders and sweeteners have been shown to cause hyper-activity and behaviour problems in infants and children, so check your labels carefully for these, too.

Contamination through your water

Some 350 different man-made chemicals can be found in tap water, and public water supplies are the source of numerous contaminants. We're not just talking about the microbes that you can encounter in some Third World countries, but also about the chemicals used in Western society to kill them. As we have seen, tap water can contain heavy metals, toxic chemicals, hormones and hormone mimics and agrochemicals. It may also contain chlorine and fluoride (see below), industrial waste, waste from toxic tips and microbes such as viruses, bacteria, parasites, algae, mould and fungi.

Tank water may be contaminated from the metal and chemicals in the roof it runs off or the tank it sits in, and by pollutants in the air the rain travels through.

Fluoride and chlorine

Both fluoride and chlorine are routinely added to most Western water supply systems. Fluoride is added to (supposedly) protect from tooth decay, and chlorine to disinfect. Chlorine is generally accepted to be a necessary evil, and many people purify their water just to get rid of its taste, but despite the controversy over whether fluoride is beneficial or harmful, many people still believe it to be a boon. Fluoride can be used as a pesticide and rat killer, and is acknowledged in many countries to be toxic. Among its effects are a possible *higher* level of dental decay (as shown in many studies) and mottled teeth. It's also been associated with cancer, genetic disorders, brittle bones, immune dysfunction, chronic fatigue, headaches, muscular weakness and spasms, gastro-intestinal problems, skin rashes, visual disturbances and disruption to enzyme production. Doesn't sound very healthy, does it? Chlorine (also used to keep swimming pools clean) is linked with heart disease, atherosclerosis, anaemia, hypertension, allergies, cancer and diabetes. Chlorine can also destroy protein and have adverse effects on skin and hair. The risk of developing cancer has been estimated in one study as being 93 per cent higher in those drinking chlorinated water. Now's the time to buy shares in a water purification business!

Making sure your water is safe

You can get your water analysed, but we suggest that the best course is to purify it. Note that this is not the same as filtering it, which can mean simply removing grit and sediment. You'll need a purifier (sometimes confusingly called a filter), which removes as many of the contaminants as possible and you'll need to purify *all* water which ends up inside you (or your baby). Boiling your water is not sufficient as it only destroys microbes, not toxins, which will be concentrated as some of the water evaporates. Of course if you ever prepare water for formula for your baby (or for any other drink for him) you must boil the water as well as purify it in order to knock off both microbes and toxins. You can take bottles of your purified water with you everywhere so you can drink a lot of it, as it helps you to gently and naturally detoxify. Since chemicals leach out of plastic, use glass bottles for water storage.

Spring water is a reasonable substitute for purified water, though it's not as reliably pure, usually comes in plastic bottles, and is very expensive if you use it for all your water needs. Mineral water is fine for an occasional drink (and very nice with a slice of lemon), but rather high in salt for frequent use.

Toxins in your home

Your home is your castle, or at least your refuge, you'll be thinking after all this gloom and doom. Maybe it's not as safe as you think, even though it's where your baby spends most of his time. Many chemicals in household products are volatile, and are easy to inhale as they become gaseous at room temperature. They get trapped in your home and concentrations have been found to peak at levels 500 times higher than outdoors. So you need to look at the chemicals that you keep in your kitchen, bathroom and laundry cupboards, not to mention the garden shed.

Spray cans, cleaning materials, air fresheners and deodorisers all contain a multitude of petrochemicals, solvents, ammonia, chlorine, phenols and other chemicals, the gases from which can be highly irritating to the mucous membranes, apart from other toxic effects. Particularly problematic are bleaches, oven cleaners and mould treatments. You should be suspicious of all preparations which have a strong fume or smell. Other problematic items include:

- synthetic or treated wool carpets (which contain many toxic chemicals)
- vinyl floor coverings
- polyester and polypropylene upholstery, bedding and clothes
- foam-filled furniture or mattresses (which contain styrenes)
- paints, varnishes, glues, stains, paint removers and wood treatments, which all contain volatile toxic compounds which are released as they dry. Paint removers also contain carbon tetrachloride, heavy metals, fungicides and insecticides. Synthetic resins and phenols are suspected carcinogens. Some contain petrochemicals.
- PVC or plastics (especially if microwaved)

- fabrics impregnated with chemical insecticides, flame retardants, crease and stain repellents
- fabrics that have been dry-cleaned (which will be impregnated with carbon tetrachloride)
- personal care products, especially those containing foaming agents such as sodium lauryl sulphate (e.g. some toothpastes) which leads to mucous membrane problems, or acetone (e.g. nail polish remover). It's best to avoid all synthetic personal care products including perfumes. (If choosing a 'natural' toothpaste, containing herbal preparations, make sure it doesn't also contain sodium lauryl sulphate.)
- detergents
- pesticides
- gas heaters and cookers (either convert to electricity or install an exhaust fan)
- furniture made from chipboard

Making your home safe

Help! Where can I live? you are probably wondering. Relax, you can stay at home. But make some changes—now. Get rid of obviously offending articles if you can. Make sure your home is well ventilated and hang dry-cleaned items out in the open air before wearing them. Grow lots of indoor plants; they freshen air, release oxygen and absorb carbon dioxide, pollutants (via the micro-organisms in the soil) and radiation. They conserve negative ions in the air (the ones that make you feel good), remove odours, smell nice and humidify the atmosphere. The best plants for these purposes are:

- *Peace Lilies*
- *Sunflowers*
- *Spider* plants
- *Bamboo*
- *Fig* trees
- *Gerberas*
- *Philodendrons*
- *Chrysanthemums*

If you can, replace carpet with tiles, unvarnished wood flooring, linoleum or rugs made from natural, untreated materials. You can choose from a wide range of 'green' cleaning products in the shops.

Health food shops tend to have more reliably non-toxic ranges than supermarkets. Listed below are some homemade alternatives which work very well.

Do-it-yourself cleaning materials
Here are a few recipes.

All purpose cleaner: 4 litres of hot water with 50 mL vinegar and 15 mL baking soda.

Dishwashing: use vinegar for heavy grease, and soap flakes instead of detergent.

Vacuuming: mix 3 cups baking soda, 4 tablespoons borax, 30 drops *Lavender* oil, 20 drops *Eucalyptus* oil, 20 drops *Lemon* oil and 20 drops *Pine* oil. Add the oils slowly, stirring the powder. Then sprinkle the mixture into the carpet, work it in and leave overnight. Vacuum. The mixture deodorises your carpet, repels fleas and smells good.

You can also use the household items listed below as cleaning agents:

- sodium bicarbonate for stainless steel, chrome, enamel
- borax for floors and tiled surfaces (but take care as borax is toxic if swallowed)
- salt for sinks, chopping boards, glass, marble, laminex
- white vinegar in hot water for cork, slate, lino, tiles, windows, mirrors, ovens, mould and deodorising
- baking soda for deodorising, spot removal, ovens, laundry, carpets, mould
- olive oil for polishing furniture and wood surfaces
- lemon juice for bleaching clothes, wood floors, toilets and deodorising

Renovating your home
Don't renovate while you're breastfeeding (or pregnant). Especially don't spruce up the nursery for your new baby. He couldn't give a tinker's cuss for the smart new decor, and would much rather be in bed with you. We've said enough about paints, solvents, glues, varnishes and synthetic materials for you to understand why.

If you must decorate or renovate, look for a supplier of environmentally friendly, non-toxic paints, glues and other products.

Toxins encountered during recreation

Golf courses are sprayed with multiple chemicals as are (to a lesser degree) many public spaces including parks. If you're a golfer, don't lick your ball to make it whizz faster. Don't put your hands in your mouth after touching surfaces that may have been sprayed. Don't swallow the water if you swim in a public pool, and shower immediately afterwards. Try to avoid visiting country areas which are heavily sprayed. If you like to garden, use organic materials, learn to love weeding and learn about companion planting to discourage weeds and pests. There are also recipes for non-toxic sprays, which can be found in the many books available on organic gardening methods.

Radiation and electro-magnetic pollution

It is not clear whether radiation and electromagnetic pollution pose a direct threat to your breast milk, but they certainly pose problems for the health of you and your baby. Ionising radiation constitutes the greatest threat, so you should avoid X-rays (which fall into this category) if at all possible. Cosmic radiation is also of the ionising variety, and each time you travel on a long-distance commercial (high-altitude) flight you are exposed to the equivalent of a full body X-ray. Other than such radical remedies as getting into the aeroplane in a lead suit (which might strain your weight allowance) or surrounding yourself with Epsom salts (which absorb some radiation but might be a bit crunchy and uncomfortable), it's quite difficult to protect yourself or your baby on a flight. There are some gadgets which you can wear which may help, and sitting away from the window is a good idea. Some herbs, *Burdock*, *Astragalus* and *Siberian Ginseng*; some nutrients, the B-complex vitamins and the antioxidants; and some homoeopathic remedies can help you and your baby to recover. But it's best to avoid flying whenever possible.

Non-ionising radiation, though not as destructive, is much more difficult to avoid. You are exposed to it through computer screens, mobile phones and microwave ovens. If you spend a lot of time in front of a computer, here are a few things you can do to minimise your exposure to radiation.

- Turn off the monitor whenever possible. The computer itself does not emit radiation and can stay on, and the more modern the monitor is, the lower the radiation. Laptops do not emit radiation, though they should not be put on the lap itself (despite the name) as this places electric fields too close to your body. Monitors are now available which use LCD screens (like a laptop's), though they are still quite expensive compared to the cathode-ray tube variety most commonly used.

- Move away from the monitor whenever possible. This means a distance of at least two metres. Remember radiation is emitted from the back and sides of monitors, as well as the front.

- Fix an anti-radiation screen to the front of the monitor. This is not the same as an anti-glare screen. These do not prevent 100 per cent of the radiation from escaping, and there will usually be leakage around the edges. The more expensive screens are more effective.

- Place some Epsom salts between yourself and the monitor, especially between the bottom of the anti-radiation screen and your body. Epsom salts absorb radiation. As they do so the crystals break down. You should replace the packet when they have become a powder. A cardboard, plastic or cotton container will not prevent the radiation reaching the crystals. You may need two packets or more to create an effective barrier.

- There are various devices available which protect against electromagnetic fields. These include a personal device to be worn on your body, devices which you can attach to the computer monitor, TV, photocopier, main cables etc, and a modulating device to plug into circuits.

- Magnetic products, which restore the body's natural static magnetism, can also be helpful. These include inner soles, mattress and seat covers.

- Grow plants in the immediate vicinity of the computer. Peace lilies and sunflowers are especially recommended.

- Take homoeopathic and herbal anti-radiation remedies. These are available from natural health practitioners.

If you use a mobile phone, here are our recommendations.

- Use your mobile phone as little as possible. It's better kept for emergencies, not regular use.

- Keep your mobile phone switched off when not in use. Remember, it attracts radiation even if you are not making a call.

- When it's switched on, keep your mobile phone at least one metre away from your body. Remember that if it's in your bag, you may still be holding it close.

- The use of hands-free kits is controversial, and though they may offer some protection, some studies seem to show that they may instead increase exposure by acting as an extra aerial. However, an aerial shield can divert the radiation away from your or your baby's body, and should be placed so that it lies between you and the aerial. Car kits can be fitted with an external aerial. (You will then need to detach the aerial on your phone.)

- These conditions also apply to cordless phones, particularly the long-range variety.

Avoiding electromagnetic pollution is more difficult if you spend much time indoors, and as the mother of a new baby this is very likely. If you live near powerlines, you might seriously consider moving. Otherwise, the best plan is to make sure your bedroom, where you and your baby probably spend a lot of your time, is as free of electromagnetic pollution as possible. Here are some tips.

- Make sure your bed is not against a wall with a fuse box or electrical appliance on the other side.

- Keep electrical gadgets turned off at the power source while you (or your baby) are asleep, as they pull current through the walls and create an electromagnetic field. This is still a problem if a pilot light is on.

- Turn off all electric blankets and water beds at the power source while you're on the bed.

- Exchange your clock radio for a wind-up or battery clock. Clock radios emit a strong local field and the illuminated digits are radioactive.

We've made the world seem a bit of a scary, dangerous place, but there *are* a lot of substances people use routinely that can affect you, your breast milk and your baby. However, there are lots of ways to avoid and combat these harmful substances, and we hope that now we have pointed them out you will adopt our recommendations to help make your breast milk as safe for your growing baby as possible. Doing this will also make you and your baby healthier in all sorts of ways—we guarantee you'll feel the difference. You'll also feel the difference if you take up the exercise program we detail in the next chapter!

Healthy exercise for better breastfeeding

If you've been committed to regular exercise before and during your pregnancy, you'll probably be keen to get back to your old routine and may even be looking forward to the liberation of exercising without that big bump in your belly. We've got a few words of caution before you start. Remember that you have just had a baby, and in traditional societies women rarely return to hard physical work straight after birth, even if they were very active right up to the time labour began. This is contrary to popular Western belief. The native woman who delivers her baby in the rice paddy and then returns immediately to back-breaking physical work is a mythical creature (or perhaps one who, unfortunately, has absolutely no other option). Most spend up to 40 days in a secluded nurturing environment where they and their babies are cared for by other women, and there are certainly good reasons for that.

Despite your desire to be physically active again, your body, especially your uterus, pelvic floor and lower back, will take a little while to regain the shape and strength that it had before you conceived. But if you've been diligent with your aerobic, strengthening and stretching routines, you'll be amazed at just how quickly and completely you get your old shape back, especially compared to women who have done no exercise at all.

All the experts recommend waiting at least six weeks after birth before you commence any serious aerobic activity, which will seem like an eternity if you're addicted to the endorphin hit that this type of exercise brings. Serious resistance or weight training should be on the back burner for about the same period of time. This gives your muscles and ligaments time to stabilise after the huge changes of pregnancy. It also gives your milk supply time to become well established. Over-exercising in the early weeks may well affect the ease with which you breastfeed.

Please don't think, as Jan did, that you know better. She waited impatiently for six weeks after the birth of her first son, but was back in training two weeks after the birth of her second, and now suffers occasional lower back problems that stem from ignoring the potential instability of that area immediately after the birth. Of course, you can start some simple pelvic floor exercises straight away and these will really pay dividends. You can continue to stretch through the early weeks as well, and walking is fine, but at all times let your body be the guide and do nothing that causes you any pain or discomfort. Immediately discontinue any activity that initiates any unusual vaginal discharge or bleeding.

However, once those six weeks have passed, it is important that you get back to some sort of exercise routine or begin one if you're not already a regular exerciser, although if you've had a Caesarean, you should check first with your obstetrician. Though your life may seem to be totally focused on nurturing your new baby (especially during the early months), it's absolutely vital that you make some time for yourself. While we're not suggesting that the time when you exercise is the only time that should be just for you, it's certainly a great place to start. The benefits include improving your overall fitness and muscular strength—and believe us, you'll need them both now that you're a mother. You'll be surprised at just how much lifting, bending, carrying and simply jumping up and down is involved in caring for a small child (not to mention the larger ones!).

If it's not possible to leave your baby with your partner while you have some time out, you can do the next best thing and take your baby with you. You can make him part of your routine. Put him in a sling or a backpack and go for a brisk walk. If you're a real enthusiast, you can even do a low impact aerobics class with your baby in his sling. He'll probably drift off to sleep, soothed by the music that he might remember from when you attended those classes during your pregnancy. Some gyms offer childminding while you're exercising. If you're not yet strong or confident enough for any of those options, invest in one of the fabulous baby carriages with giant pneumatic tyres. Pushing your baby in one of these can provide a great aerobic work-out.

THE BENEFITS OF EXERCISE

Once your milk supply is well established you can be sure that exercise won't affect it in any way. Although it has been suggested that the production of lactic acid might change the taste of your milk, we've never seen any definitive studies indicating this to be the case, and even if it does we think it unlikely that your baby will find it off-putting. Certainly none of our babies did. So regular exercise while you're breastfeeding should only confer benefits.

Better delivery of oxygen and nutrients

Aerobic exercise, which includes power walking, swimming, cycling and jogging, gives your lungs and heart a work-out. This means they will work more efficiently and your whole body will benefit from their improved function. There'll be a more efficient delivery of oxygen and of essential nutrients to all your tissues including your breast milk. Beware of exercising in toxic environments such as swimming pools treated with chemicals and roads that have heavy traffic. You might want to wear a mask if you can't avoid walking or exercising near main roads.

More efficient healing

Because of the improvement in your circulation, labial tears and grazes will heal quickly and so will any surgical wounds such as an episiotomy or Caesarean incision.

Better bowel and kidney function

Aerobic exercise improves peristalsis (that's the movement of your gut), which means you'll be less likely to suffer from constipation. Of course, while you're exercising you'll also be drinking lots of purified water, which is a simple and safe way to flush toxins from your body. Good bowel and kidney function are helpful for keeping breast milk free of accumulated toxicity and safe for your baby.

Retention of calcium

Aerobic exercise will help your body to use up any excess kilojoules that you might have gained during your pregnancy, and if the exercise is weight-bearing—like walking, jogging, cycling or taking part in aerobics classes (but not swimming)—this will help increase your bone density because more calcium is retained by your body. This means a reduced risk of osteoporosis later in your life (long after your child-bearing years are over), but while you're breastfeeding it's particularly important that the maximum amount of calcium is retained in your bones. It's important to maintain the integrity of your bones during breastfeeding because there's a drain on your calcium stores at this time (which may also have been depleted during pregnancy).

More energy, sounder sleep

Regular aerobic exercise means you'll have improved stamina and endurance. This is a great bonus when you're carrying your baby in a sling or backpack. Contrary to what you might expect, you'll also experience less fatigue, you'll feel less stressed, and you'll sleep better with regular exercise. Breastfeeding will be easier when you're relaxed and your milk supply will be assured if you're sleeping well.

Enhanced feelings of wellbeing

Regular exercise is renowned for its positive effects on mood. This is due to the production of endorphins, which are natural mood enhancers. These chemicals are also an integral part of breastfeeding, contributing to the sense of wellbeing that is so vital if the breastfeeding experience is to be satisfying and long-term.

Supple body, reduced stiffness

Stretching is a great way to relax and reduce tension. It will also increase your flexibility so you will be able to experience the full range of motion for which your body was designed without experiencing any stiffness. Improved flexibility means it is much less likely that you will sustain an injury with all the bending, lifting and carrying that comes with simply being a mother. This is important at any time, but particularly when you're breastfeeding and carrying your baby in a sling, shifting him from side to side while lying down and accommodating his gymnastic feeding positions as he grows older.

Strong pelvic floor muscles

Strong pelvic floor muscles mean that you won't suffer from incontinence. More on this later in the chapter.

Positive preparation for your next pregnancy

While another pregnancy shouldn't be on your agenda for a good while yet—we recommend at least two years between pregnancies—it's never too soon to start thinking about your preconception health care. A regular exercise routine is an integral part of preparing positively for another baby.

HOW TO EXERCISE SAFELY

So there's absolutely no doubt that exercise has lots of benefits for you, and indirectly for your breastfeeding baby. An ideal program would incorporate aerobic and resistance exercise as well as stretching, but if you have any questions or specific health concerns you should consult a fitness centre, personal trainer or health practitioner. You can safely start with some gentle pelvic floor exercises and some simple stretching (see later in this chapter) very shortly after the birth. When you're ready you can move on to something more strenuous, and we'll describe some suitable routines a little further on. Whatever the level of your exertions, however, there are a few things to remember before you begin.

- Warm up.

- Take it easy at first.

☆ Slow down if necessary.

☆ Stay cool and keep well hydrated (drink plenty of purified water).

☆ Choose an exercise that is comfortable, calming and cushioning if your pelvic floor muscles are still weak, or if you've undergone a Caesarean.

☆ Avoid rapid changes in direction and bouncing during exercise.

☆ Always try to maintain correct posture.

☆ Don't hold your breath; breathe continuously while exercising.

☆ Cool down; stretch out.

☆ Never overstretch; control the movement.

☆ Never exercise through any pain or discomfort.

☆ Consult your doctor if you experience any unusual symptoms.

START WITH YOUR PELVIC FLOOR MUSCLES

If you've had a vaginal birth, your pelvic floor muscles have just had the work-out of their lives. You may have worked at strengthening them before you went into labour, but whether you did or not, now is the time to get them back into tip-top shape. And it's definitely well worth the effort.

If you've wondered why women with children prefer walking to running and why they always choose low-impact aerobic classes, the chances are it's because their pelvic floor muscles are very weak. These muscles, which were probably already weak when the women gave birth, were traumatised by their babies' entrance into the world, and have been sadly neglected ever since.

A weak pelvic floor means incontinence. You will wet your pants when you jump or run and sometimes even when you laugh or cough or sneeze. This is definitely not a good look! So you need to know how to strengthen those muscles, and you must continue to strengthen them, especially after your baby is born.

Your pelvic floor muscles are a sling-like band that surrounds and forms the base of the vagina, anus and urethra. The muscles support all the abdominal contents and your baby passes through them as he is born. It will help you to identify them if you try this exercise.

Next time you urinate, try to stop the flow in mid-stream, then, after a moment or two, relax the muscles—you have just exercised your pelvic floor. We don't recommend you do the exercise each time you urinate— just until you get the hang of contracting and releasing.

You can start the following pelvic floor (Kegel) exercise just 24 hours after giving birth. Lie face down on the floor (or on a bed) with your arms at your sides. Tighten and relax your pelvic floor muscles. Repeat 10 times.

After three or four days, you can vary this exercise by lifting one leg at a time and tightening the pelvic floor muscles as you do so. This creates the effect of squeezing out a sponge and initiating a fresh flow of blood to the area. If you've had an episiotomy, you'll find this speeds up the rate of healing.

Now that you are familiar with the sensation, you can repeat this exercise whenever you like. You can do the exercise when you're sitting or standing too and it's one of the few exercises that you can do any time, any place. Just think, nobody need ever know! Try to increase the number of times you contract and release your pelvic floor, and also increase the time for which you hold each contraction. Repeat the exercise at least five times every hour and hold each contraction for at least five seconds.

You can try another version of this exercise. Think of the pelvic floor muscles as a lift. Take the lift up several floors and be sure to stop at each floor. Then take the lift down, stopping again at each floor. When you reach the ground floor, continue to the basement. To do this you must release your pelvic floor muscles completely. This is what you do when you urinate or empty your bowels and it's how you use those muscles in the second stage of labour.

STRETCHING FOR FLEXIBILITY

Simple stretching exercises can be begun two or three days after you've given birth. Doing these stretches regularly means that your muscles will be supple and ready for activity and movement (and there's plenty of that ahead with your young baby). You should always stretch at the end of every aerobic exercise session too. We have included below some stretching exercises for your whole body. Hold each stretch for at least 30 seconds.

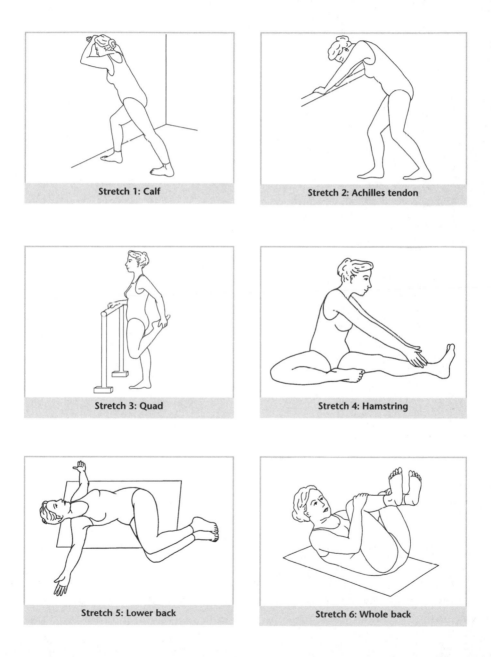

Stretch 1: Calf

Stretch 2: Achilles tendon

Stretch 3: Quad

Stretch 4: Hamstring

Stretch 5: Lower back

Stretch 6: Whole back

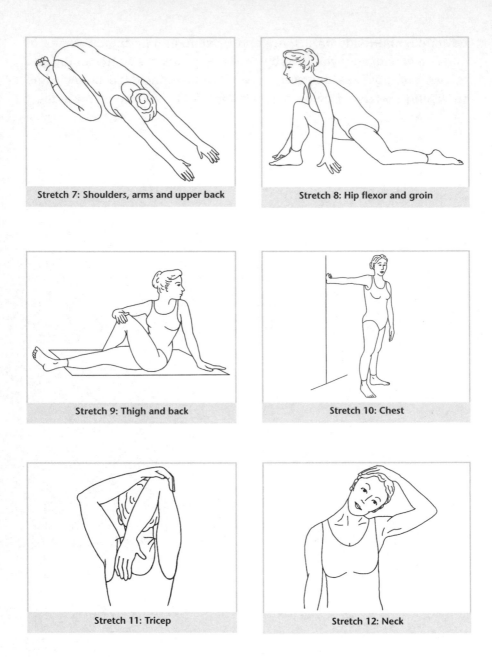

Stretch 7: Shoulders, arms and upper back

Stretch 8: Hip flexor and groin

Stretch 9: Thigh and back

Stretch 10: Chest

Stretch 11: Tricep

Stretch 12: Neck

YOGA

Even if you were a dedicated aerobic afficionado before your pregnancy, in your new role as a breastfeeding mother you might prefer the
calm, inward centred approach of yoga to the running–jumping types

of exercise. Regular yoga practice confers lots of significant benefits. One of the most important of these is the ability to put your body and mind into a very relaxed state. Yoga exercises will also help strengthen back, abdominal and pelvic muscles after pregnancy and childbirth.

If you're a complete novice, you might prefer to attend yoga classes where a qualified yoga teacher can guide you. In a structured class, the correct postures can be easily learned. However, we describe below some simple yoga poses that anyone can do with complete safety. When you're practising at home it's wise to build the time spent in each posture gradually. Even if you don't hold the posture for the maximum time, any time spent in a posture will still be beneficial. Daily practice is recommended for best results. You can keep your baby right beside you while you're practising and this is an advantage for mothers who wouldn't otherwise be able to exercise.

Baddha Konasana (Supta): The cobbler pose

Sit on the floor with the soles of your feet together, heels as close as possible to your perineum (that's the area between your anus and vulva), with a folded blanket under your feet. Press your toes open against a wall. Then lie back with a folded blanket supporting your head and neck if you wish. Initially, you should try to hold this pose for 2 minutes, building to 5, 10, then 15 minutes. When you're ready to get up, use your left hand to manually lift the left knee over to the right knee and allow your body to roll to the right, finally coming up on your hands and knees.

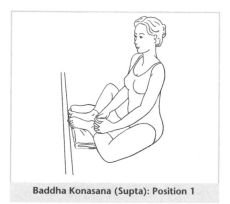

Baddha Konasana (Supta): Position 1

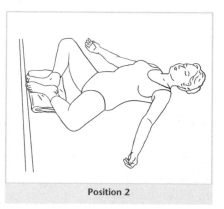

Position 2

Virabhadrasana II:
The second warrior pose

This is a standing posture and very useful for increasing strength which you'll need for carrying your new baby. Stand with your back against a wall for support. Place your feet about a metre apart, pointing your right foot away from you and with the left turned in slightly. With your right knee in line with the second toe of your right foot, slowly bend the right knee until it forms a right angle. Hold your arms out straight against the wall at shoulder height, and keep the back leg strong with the knee pulled up. Build to 30 seconds. Come up slowly, keeping the right knee in line with the second right toe on the way up to avoid knee strain. Repeat on the other side.

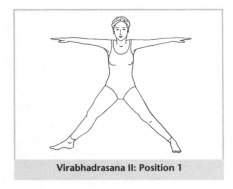

Virabhadrasana II: Position 1

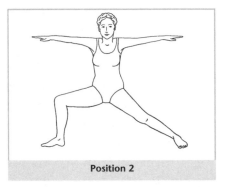

Position 2

Upavista Konasana

Position a chair in front of you, then sit on the floor with your legs straight and opened comfortably (but not as wide as they will go). Press your heels away, push into your feet, keep your toes turned up. Use the chair to keep your body upright. Aim to get your thigh bones flat on the floor. Build up to 3 minutes.

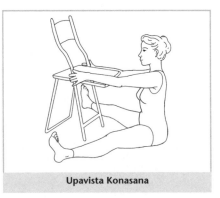

Upavista Konasana

Virasana (Supta)

Kneel with your feet apart, buttocks between your feet with a folded blanket beneath them. Make sure your feet are facing straight back. When this posture becomes comfortable, lean back, either against a chair, or on folded blankets, bolsters or supportive cushions. Build gradually to 10 minutes. Come up slowly.

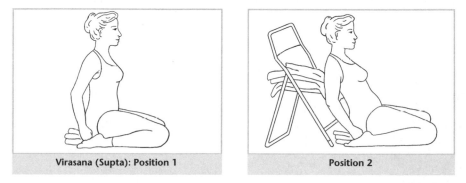

Virasana (Supta): Position 1   **Position 2**

When you feel comfortable with these poses, you might like to vary your routine by including some additional postures.

Backward bending

Stand with your feet about shoulder-width apart and place your hands on your hips. Keep your feet pointing forwards. Bend back slowly. Hold for 30 seconds, then return slowly to the starting position.

Forward bending

From backward bending you can gently move into forward bending. Keep your knees slightly bent, spread your legs apart, relax your head and shoulders and just hang down.

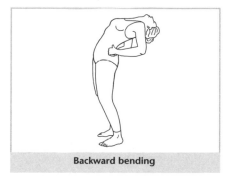

Backward bending

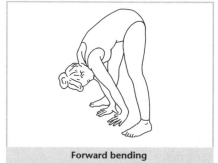

Forward bending

Half headstand

Headstands and shoulderstands are very helpful and rest your back and lower abdominals and the muscles in your legs. However, you shouldn't attempt these poses if you're a novice. Instead, try a half headstand, using a wall for support. With your head resting on a folded blanket and your shoulders against the wall, take one leg off the ground and hold for 30 seconds. Increase the time you hold the pose as you gain in confidence.

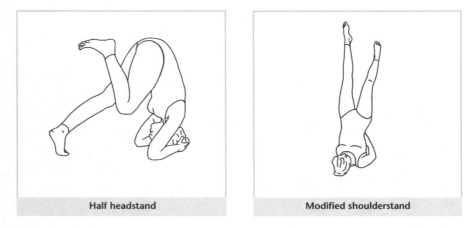

Half headstand   Modified shoulderstand

Modified shoulderstand

This is a great way to take the weight off legs that might be tired from carrying your baby. Lying with your buttocks against the wall, and using your hands for support, stretch your legs up until they are straight. Then practise taking one leg at a time off the wall.

Forward bend (from the sitting position)

Sit with your legs apart. Bend forward from the hips, keeping your spine straight and spreading your thighs. Don't hunch your shoulders or back. You may be able to hold onto your toes as your flexibility increases.

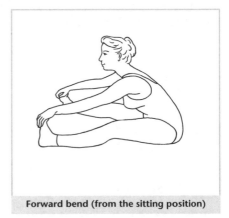

Forward bend (from the sitting position)

Crescent moon

Kneel on the floor then step forward with one leg. Placing your hands on your forward knee for support, bend back slowly and carefully. Relax your head.

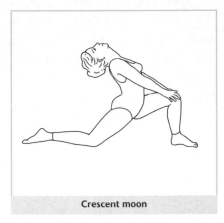

Crescent moon

Butterfly

You may have practised this posture already in Baddha Konasana Supta. Lie with your buttocks and feet against the wall. Keep the soles of your feet together and let your knees drop down to the sides. You can press down gently on your knees with your hands.

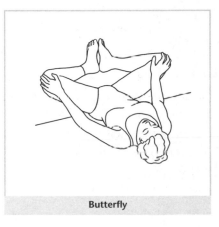

Butterfly

Spinal twist

Sit cross-legged on the floor. Place your hand on the opposite knee and the other hand on the floor behind you. Twist gently in the direction of the hand that's behind you. Repeat on the other side.

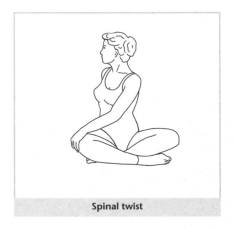

Spinal twist

Standing spinal twist

Stand with your legs crossed, then with arms outspread twist in the direction of the front leg. Repeat on the other side.

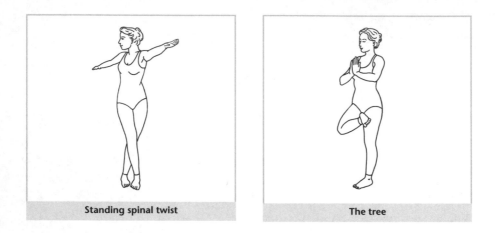

Standing spinal twist

The tree

The tree

Standing positions strengthen your legs and this one requires good balance too. Begin by putting the sole of one foot on the ankle bone of the other and with your hands in prayer position hold the pose. If you're an advanced student you can rest the sole of your foot on the inner thigh of the other leg.

Modified abdominal corpse pose

This is a resting pose. Lying on your front, supporting your head on one or both arms, draw up your legs one by one. Hold each leg in position for a minute or two.

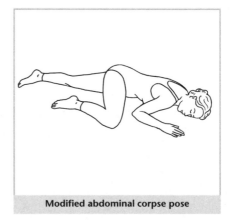

Modified abdominal corpse pose

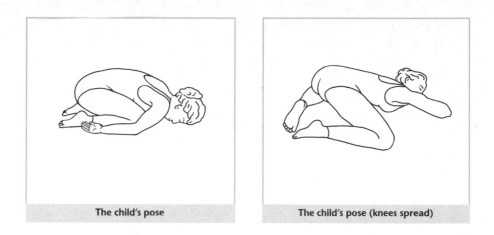

The child's pose

The child's pose (knees spread)

The child's pose

This resting position can be alternated with all the previous positions. Kneel with your knees together on the floor then sink back so that your buttocks touch your heels. Reach your arms straight out in front of you, palms turned down. You can vary this position by splaying your knees out to the sides and pushing your chest towards the floor.

MUSCLE-STRENGTHENING EXERCISES

It goes without saying that strong muscles are important for a new mother, particularly a breastfeeding one. There's lots of work for those muscles to do; not least of their jobs is to support the extra weight of your breasts. And strong back, shoulder, buttock, abdominal and leg muscles are vital if you're planning to carry your baby attached to your body in some sort of sling (or in a backpack when he's older) for a considerable part of the day. He'll certainly be happiest when he's close to you, so it's in both your interests to strengthen those muscles. And, trust us, the need to be strong doesn't stop once your baby becomes mobile. The extra lifting and carrying, which is considerable, continues for years (probably forever—we'll let you know).

If you attend a fitness centre, you can ask a qualified instructor to show you specific resistant exercises that are suitable for a new mother. These can be done using either free weights or the fixed weight machines. However you might prefer to do your muscle building in private. If this is the case, Jan's business partner has the answer for you.

The TUBETRAIN exercise system is easy to use and works every muscle group. It's also completely portable and comes complete with instructional brochure and workout video. Alternatively, you can purchase a small set of hand weights, or you can substitute two unbreakable bottles filled with water and use these as weights. Below are some examples of muscle-strengthening exercises. Repeat each exercise 10 times, then have a rest for 60 seconds. This is called one set. Repeat the sequence. As you become stronger you can increase the number of repetitions and the number of sets you perform at each session.

Abdomen

Lie on your back, feet flat on the floor close to your buttocks. Support your head with your hands, making sure you don't pull up on your neck. Lift your head and shoulders and twist to the left. Return to the starting position and repeat, twisting to the right.

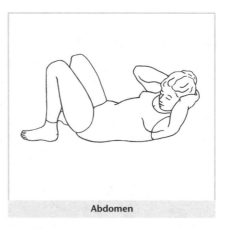

Abdomen

Legs

Start with your feet shoulder-width apart. Take a good step back on to the ball of one foot. Looking straight ahead, bend your front knee and drop your hips until your thigh is parallel to the floor. Return to the starting position by pushing up with your front leg. Repeat for the other leg.

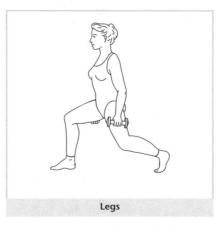

Legs

Arms

Stand with your feet slightly apart and elbows locked into your sides. Curl the weights towards your shoulder, contracting your bi-ceps. Release slowly, keeping your elbows fixed by your side as you go. If you prefer, you can alternate arms.

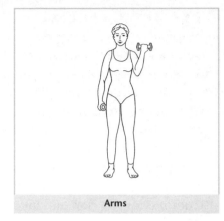

Arms

Chest

Stand with your feet shoulder-width apart. With your hands close to your chest, at about nipple level, and with elbows high, push the weights away from your body. Return slowly to the starting position.

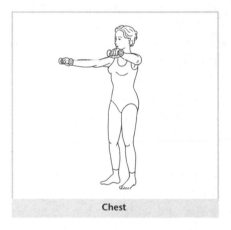

Chest

Shoulders

Stand with feet apart (you may be more comfortable with one foot slightly in front of the other). Lift your elbows sideways to shoulder height, keeping your arms bent. At the finish position your hands should be slightly lower than your elbows and tilted so that your little fingers are slightly higher than your thumbs.

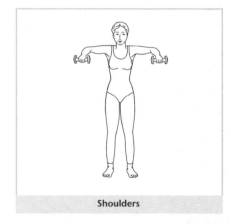

Shoulders

Aerobic exercise

A regular aerobic exercise routine should involve a minimum of 30 minutes of aerobic activity at each session. You should try for at least three sessions per week. If you are already physically fit, then your body will have developed physiological responses to allow you to cope well with the circulatory and respiratory changes that occur during exercise. However, these mechanisms won't be quite so well adapted if you've never exercised at all, and any strenuous activity to which you are unaccustomed could be stressful. Therefore, if you're breastfeeding and exercising seriously for the first time, check with a health practitioner before you start and take things very gently to begin with.

The best sort of aerobic exercise is one where you can take your baby along, e.g. in a sling (later a backpack) while you walk briskly. You might prefer to put him in one of those fabulous buggies and walk or jog. If he's involved, he'll get a very important message—life is about movement and activity. His position receptors will be stimulated at the same time—and that's important for his brain development.

Even if you're feeling quite tired from attending to the needs of your new baby, if you begin (or continue) an exercise program, you'll probably find your energy levels pick up quite a lot. Your circulation will improve and the better delivery of nutrients will make you feel more energetic. The endorphins that are produced will give you a general feeling of well-being, and you'll sleep more soundly too. But whether you decide on a swim or a walk or a bike ride, just start off gently and, over the coming weeks, gradually build up to a more sustained level of activity. Remember that there's no need to push to achieve a pre-pregnancy level of training and remember to keep well hydrated (10–12 glasses of purified water daily, more in hot weather) and always drink before you become thirsty.

To wean or not to wean?

Let's stop for a minute and recall some of the advantages of breast-feeding for your baby. He gets nutrients in the most easily assimilated form and factors important for the development of his eyes and his brain (which develops at a great rate for the first three years of his life). He gets immunity from a host of diseases and protection against allergies. Breastfeeding promotes correct facial and dental develop-ment, ensures that all his senses are stimulated appropriately and improves his fine motor co-ordination. Your baby also receives comfort, feelings of security and an enhanced sense of his value as an indi-vidual. He needs all of these things for more than just the first few months of his life if he is to achieve optimal physical, mental and emotional development.

But the advantages aren't just for your baby. You get an effective method of child-spacing, a food supply that is never-ending and absolutely hassle-free and an effective tranquilliser as well. You get an enhanced sense of self-worth and a wonderful level of intimacy with your baby. You definitely need all of these things for the first few years of his life for your optimal physical and emotional wellbeing. So there are many excellent reasons for you to continue to breastfeed until your child decides for himself that he has had enough.

WHY NOT LET YOUR CHILD DECIDE?

If you really feel that your child will never be finished with your breasts, rest assured that, contrary to the opinions of friends and relatives, one day he will wean himself. The day will definitely come when he simply won't be interested anymore. Despite dire predictions that we would both be offering our breasts at the university gates, all our boys weaned themselves in their own good time. However, Francesca's first son was old enough to be reaching for Playboy from the newsagent's stand while calling out 'Tit! tit!', and Jan's boys were eased into their first days of school with a quick breastfeed. But we know that those years of breast-feeding paid off because all our sons are not only exceptionally healthy and bright, but they are very secure and loving individuals as well.

Each child has his own timetable for weaning so let him follow it if you possibly can. Lynne McTaggart, the editor of What Doctors Don't Tell You and Natural Parent, sums it up succinctly. 'I only feel comfortable taking my cue from nature. Virtually every tribal culture tends to feed partially for several years. When children no longer need it, they stop. Perhaps we ought to ask the experts on this issue. Only three-year-olds need apply!'

A NATURAL PROGRESSION

Traditional societies usually nursed until a child (no longer a baby by then) said 'Enough!' This could have been anywhere into the child's third, fourth or fifth year. One day, that child simply decided that he no longer needed the comfort of breastfeeding and as easily as that he was weaned. No fuss, no tears, just a perfectly natural progression to his next stage of development. In animal species, it's the more skilful groups that have the longest period of breastfeeding so that should tell us something about the importance of prolonged nursing for the human species.

If we accept that traditional societies fed their children for a number of years, it should also be apparent that they often fed more than one child at a time. The lactational amenorrhoea that results from unre-stricted breastfeeding (particularly unrestricted night-time nursing) would last up to two years, making a sibling a possibility about nine

PROLONGED BREASTFEEDING

If you're committed to a prolonged breastfeeding relationship, here are some tips to ensure that you can feed for as long as your child wants to.

- Attend to your diet and your supplementation regimen just as carefully as you did during the preconception period. Take your supplements as described in Chapter 5 and continue for the whole period of breastfeeding. (Of course we have to question why you'd ever stop.)
- If you're following a vegetarian diet, make absolutely certain that you're getting adequate protein and in the right combinations (see Chapter 5), and be scrupulous with your supplementation, making sure that vitamins B12 and iron are included.
- Remember that breast milk provides comfort as well as food and drink.
- Use your breast as a pacifier. Throw away plastic dummies. A dummy will reduce your baby's desire to suck, and it may contain phthalates, which are toxic hormone disruptors.
- Feed your baby on demand day and night. If he has 20 feeds a day in the early weeks, don't despair. Nothing stays the same and if you attend to those needs then, he'll make fewer demands on you when he's older.
- Until the introduction of solids (see elsewhere in this chapter), offer nothing other than breast milk, even in hot weather.
- Introduce solid food only when your baby reaches for it from your plate.
- Let your child initiate the weaning process. Be prepared for him to be a very mobile (and possibly articulate) toddler before this happens.
- Expect to be free of menstrual periods for a considerable time (years for some women, particularly older ones) if you practise this method of completely unrestricted breastfeeding.
- If your menstrual cycle resumes, you may find that your baby shows less inclination to nurse when you are either menstruating or ovulating, as the taste of the milk can change at these times.
- Rest assured that despite all indications to the contrary, one day your baby will bypass your breasts for more interesting activities (and there might even be a few years' grace before he finds breasts fascinating again). Both Jan and Francesca and many other mums who have breastfed their children until they weaned themselves have had to cope with being undressed in public by a demanding toddler. Never fear, we're sure you will handle all this with the grace and equanimity that the love for your child bestows.

> ⚮ Don't despair if your child's first teeth show some decay. While the typical pattern of 'bottle mouth' is due to the child going to bed while sucking on a bottle of Ribena or other sweet drink, a child who has had the benefits of prolonged breastfeeding (especially if he likes to fall asleep with the nipple in his mouth) may exhibit a similar pattern of decay. Remember these are 'milk' teeth and they're probably called that for a very good reason.

months later, just shortly before the first child's third birthday. Interestingly, studies show that the ideal for child-spacing is at least two years. This gives the mother a chance to restore her nutritional status and ensures that the first child has had adequate nurturing and nursing.

So conceivably (no pun intended) the mother relying on breastfeeding for contraception, who conceived as soon as she was ovulating again, could give birth to her new baby before her first was weaned. She might then continue to feed them both for a year or two before the older child weaned himself. Clearly, today this would take a superior level of physical health, emotional stamina and commitment. How many women have you seen nursing both a three-year-old and a newborn?

While present cultural and social expectations have a lot to do with the fact that this is a rare exception, it's worth remembering that it was often the norm and that the physical and emotional resources of those women were clearly up to the task.

Today, of course, lifestyles are very different and prolonged breastfeeding and tandem nursing occur less and less frequently. Women choose to restrict the period of breastfeeding, they elect to have their children very close together or they make a decision to return to work. They may simply decide that a toddler who lifts their shirt in search of sustenance in the middle of a busy supermarket is not an option for them. While we don't believe that any of these choices mean that you have to wean your baby (or your toddler) completely, we also accept that the choice is a very individual one. But remember, the World Health Organisation now recommends breastfeeding for a minimum period of two years. It should be obvious from all the benefits of breastfeeding that we've already outlined that we heartily endorse that recommendation, and would encourage you to breastfeed for just as long as your child wants to continue.

However, you may need or wish to wean your child earlier, so we'll tell you how to go about it to minimise your and your baby's physical and emotional discomfort.

IF YOU NEED TO WEAN A BABY

If you really need to wean your baby, there are some important things to consider. First, and you may think this is too obvious to mention, don't start to wean him (or start him on solids) while he is sick. Secondly, take your time. After all, weaning means 'accustom infant to food other than human milk'. The key word is 'accustom' which is a very different thing from 'instant withdrawal'. If at all possible, continue to nurse your baby for at least some of the time. Even if he's not getting very much milk, he will probably still enjoy suckling at your breast.

Gradual weaning is best

It will be easier if you eliminate feeds one at a time. The first to go is often a feed in the late afternoon or early evening when your milk supply may be low and you may be tired and distracted. If you've been feeding ad lib, it's really more a question of reducing the number of times your baby nurses during the day. It might, for example, be possible to distract him with other activities in the morning, when he's fresh. But whatever schedule you choose for reducing the frequency of feeding, the bed time feed will probably be the last to go. However, don't feel you need to keep to any rigid plan, and be sensitive to your baby's needs—let him call the shots.

Gradual weaning is easier on your baby's digestive system, and avoids reactions such as stomach-ache which can result if he isn't given time to adapt to substitute milks or new foods. He also has to learn new ways of receiving food and drink, and adapt to a cup or a bottle. If you have breastfed for long enough not to need to resort to formula or other milk substitutes, there is no need to use a bottle. If weaning occurs after your baby is 9 or 10 months old, you can use a cup for fluids, as he will have less need to suck, and there are many spill-proof baby beakers on the market. If your baby still needs to suck, perhaps you have weaned too early. Remember, you can still offer the breast for comfort long after he's stopped relying on it for food.

If you take your time weaning your baby, there will also be fewer risks for you. Your breasts will naturally produce less milk as your baby sucks less. If you stop suddenly, your breasts may become engorged with milk, which can be very uncomfortable. Although the engorgement will itself put pressure on the alveoli (the milk-producing ducts) and eventually dry up your supply, there is a danger of mastitis developing. Another advantage of a gradual approach is that you will retain more of the fatty tissue in your breasts. After weaning, it's common for your breasts to be much smaller than they were before conception, though this fat deficit is usually replaced within a year.

Suppressing lactation

You may find that your milk supply dries up quite easily. Some women, however, especially those with a very plentiful milk supply, need to use specific remedies to suppress lactation and avoid engorgement. Once, this was achieved by binding the breasts tightly. Although we certainly don't recommend this approach, it's a good idea to avoid stimulating your breasts through touch, or by expressing milk. Other less than ideal methods include limiting your fluid intake, or putting something that tastes nasty on your nipples. Since we're great believers in being well hydrated at all times, we certainly don't endorse the first approach, and the second just ruins your baby's last experience of what has been his life support and closest connection with you.

Until recently the medical treatment was to give oestrogen in tablet form as it reduces prolactin levels. This is not done anymore because of the adverse effects. These days the medical approach is to prescribe bromocriptine, a drug which suppresses prolactin production, through its action on the pituitary. Painkillers are sometimes prescribed, as well as antibiotics if the situation deteriorates into engorgement or mastitis. To avoid using these drugs, there are natural remedies listed below.

- Sage is the herb usually used to dry up breast milk. Red Sage is best, though garden sage will do if that's all that's available. Drink a cup of sage tea (infusion) 3–4 times daily until the milk flow has stopped. This may take several days. Other herbs which may be useful are Bugleweed and Peppermint. (See Appendix 5 for how to make an infusion.)

- Jasmine flowers have been shown in a clinical trial to be as effective as bromocriptine for engorgement and lactation suppression. In this trial, 50 cm of stringed flowers were attached to the breast with sticky tape. Jasmine has a lowering effect on prolactin, and may also be used as an essential oil. Rub some on your breasts (but make sure your baby doesn't suck it), put it in your bath, in a burner or an inhaler.

- The homoeopathic remedy to use is Lac caninum. Take a single dose of the 200 c potency, and repeat 2–3 days later if the milk is still coming.

- The higher doses of vitamin B6 can suppress prolactin and lactation. Take 500 mg daily (in the short term only), and watch for side effects such as tingling or numbness in the fingertips, toes or upper lip.

- To help you get through any feelings of loss or sadness when you stop feeding, try the Bach flower remedy Walnut. This is the remedy for all times of transition and change. A few drops under your baby's tongue could help him too.

After weaning, you may still have small amounts of milk in your breasts, especially if your baby suckles occasionally for comfort. This is quite normal for several weeks or even months after the last feed.

Choosing a formula

Below are some of the things you might want to consider if you have to choose an alternative to prolonged breastfeeding.

- You might consider alternating two or three different formulae or milks (such as goat's, soya and rice). That way, your baby will be less likely to develop an allergy. Be prepared to change to a different formula if he exhibits any signs that indicate intolerance (see later in this chapter).

- Try to avoid cow's milk and formulae based on cow's milk as it is a very common allergen. (Note, however, that infant cow's milk allergy is usually due to the protein or phenolic factors in the milk, and not to lactose intolerance, which is unusual in babies. Under the age of 3, babies have a plentiful supply of lactase, which is necessary for the digestion of the lactose in breast milk. As they get older, especially in non-Caucasian races, the supply of lactase diminishes, and lactose intolerance becomes more of a problem, as it can during bouts of diarrhoea, even in a breastfed baby. The protein molecules in cow's milk are much larger than those of human milk and are difficult for your baby to digest. Cow's milk or formulae based on cow's milk given in the first few months of a baby's life may also be linked to the later onset of diabetes.

- Do not use soya milk extensively. The isoflavones, including genistein and equol, which are found in soy demonstrate toxicity in oestrogen-sensitive tissues and in the thyroid. This potential for soy to interfere with the formation of your baby's hormone receptor sites is shown by the case of a girl raised exclusively on soy who menstruated at the age of 5, and another who developed pubic hair when only 8. In the United States, where nearly 25 per cent of babies are fed soya formulae, 1 per cent show signs of puberty by the age of 3 years, such as breast development or pubic hair. By age 8 this figure rises to 15 per cent for white American girls and 50 per cent for African–American girls. A number of authorities now suggest avoiding soy for the first two years of your child's life.

- Another concern with soy is the presence of aluminium and phytates. Aluminium levels are higher in non-organically grown soya products, and phytates are present in the non-fermented forms of soya (such as beans and milk). Soy is traditionally used in Asian cultures only in its fermented forms, which don't contain phytates. These have a possible blocking action on the absorption of proteins and other nutrients such as calcium, magnesium, copper, iron and zinc. Phytates have also been shown to cause delayed growth in children.

- Goat's milk formula is an alternative option, and one West Australian study shows it to be free of chemical contamination, even when the goats were not organically fed. The protein molecule in goat's milk is much closer in size to that of human milk compared to cow's milk.

❋ Rice milk is a reasonably good source of protein, though not as good as an animal milk, and it has little fatty content, so you should add half a teaspoon of flaxseed oil to each feed and shake well.

❋ The addition of lactobacilli, extracted from whey, to a baby's bottle will help your baby's immunity, since the whey has a high level of immunoglobulin and antibodies, just like colostrum. This will also help to prevent constipation, often a problem in bottle-fed infants.

❋ Make up feeds exactly according to the instructions.

❋ Always use purified water to make up formula feeds. This is an additional requirement to boiling, as boiling only kills bacteria and does not eliminate toxins.

❋ Do not microwave formula or substitute milk as microwaving changes the molecular structure of food, destroying nutrients.

❋ Discard any unused formula.

❋ Use glass bottles. PVC products (those with the figure '3' inside the recycling symbol) should be avoided. PVC contains phthalates and may also contain the toxic metals cadmium and lead. Phthalates are organic products used to plasticise or soften the PVC and can migrate into the formula from the plastic. Phthalates are hormone disrupters and have been linked to liver, kidney and testicular cancer. Since the discovery of these adverse effects about fifteen years ago, PVC has been made much safer, and other, less toxic alternatives have been developed, but it's still a good idea to use glass containers whenever possible. If plastic is the only option, choose PET, HDPE, LDPE or PP products.

INTRODUCING SOLIDS

No matter when you choose to wean, you'll have to start your baby on suitable solid foods at an appropriate age. Despite what your family or friends might tell you, there are absolutely no benefits in giving your baby solids before he is 6 months old. Until he can sit up he will find it difficult to digest solids, as gravity has a part to play in the passage of food down the gut. The age at which he starts on solid food isn't a measure of his intelligence or any other developmental milestone, and it's a myth that giving solids will encourage him to sleep through the night. Rather, several health problems can result if you start him on solids too early. Premature introduction of solid foods can cause kidney problems, which can lead to dehydration and have serious consequences for his health. The absorption of iron (best provided by breast milk), can be compromised, possibly leading to anaemia. The risk of developing coeliac disease is increased if gluten-containing cereals (wheat, rye, barley and oats) are introduced too early.

Your baby's digestive system matures slowly and many of the enzymes required for digestion are absent for many months. Before 6 months of age your baby's gut is still permeable and foreign proteins that are a result of incomplete digestion of food can be absorbed through the intestinal mucosa. These foreign proteins go on to cause allergies and intolerances to that food. It's no coincidence that the most common allergenic foods—dairy products, wheat, eggs and oranges—are those that clinic sisters previously recommended as 'first foods'.

After about 6 months (but the time will vary quite a bit and it may be closer to 8 or 9 months) your baby makes his own secretory IgA which coats the intestines and stops the absorption of foreign proteins. Therefore the recommendation of experts (including the World Health Organisation) is for no solids before 6 months. Further, along with a lot of experts working in the field of clinical ecology, we recommend that you wait until 12 months before you introduce any of the major allergens to your baby's diet. This will fly in the face of the feeding practices of most of your friends and their babies, so be prepared to stick to your beliefs, especially if there's any history of allergy in your family or your partner's.

Reaching for food

At about 6 months most babies lose their tongue-thrust reflex. Before this, if you try to introduce solid foods, especially with a spoon, you may find that your baby simply pushes the food out of his mouth. Many mothers mistakenly assume this is because he doesn't like the taste of the food, and try another, and another, and so on. Also around this time he will usually have some teeth and will become interested in what's on your plate. We think his interest should be the sign that he is ready for some sort of solid food. However, it's not uncommon for a fully breastfed baby to be quite a bit older before he starts to reach for your lunch or dinner. Rest assured that he's still getting adequate nutrition at your breast and he'll start to eat when the time is right.

Finger foods

Since your baby is the one doing the reaching, we recommend that once he shows an interest you let him select the food and handle it by himself. You can save yourself a lot of extra work—cooking, pureeing, mashing and straining—by giving him finger foods with which to experiment, and his co-ordination will improve at the same time that you're saving time and energy. Your baby will love the opportunity to feed himself and if you allow him to make his own choices he's much less likely to exhibit odd fads and fancies. Forget about the mess he makes when he starts to feed himself, put some newspaper under his highchair and let him help himself. Obviously some foods are better suited than others to being picked up in the fingers; you'll soon work out what he can and can't manage.

Remember that a lot of his early feeding experiences are nothing more than experimentation. And he'll be experimenting with more than new tastes—texture is also important, and he'll probably be interested in how food feels rubbed into his hair, thrown at the cat, squashed through his fingers, and offered to you, as well as how it feels and tastes in his mouth. (Don't worry, he'd make just as much mess if he was blowing raspberries with fruit puree presented to him on a spoon.) In this phase, continue to give him a breastfeed before you introduce him to a new food. That way you can be sure he's still receiving adequate nutrition.

First foods

It's interesting to look at older cultures in which the babies were fed nothing but breast milk for anything from one to two years. The first food that these babies were offered had been thoroughly chewed and therefore drenched in their mothers' saliva (and digestive enzymes). This overcame the problem of the babies' immature digestive systems.

If you draw the line at pre-masticating your baby's food, you could start by introducing low-reactive fruits such as pear and papaya. But don't overdose your baby on fruit. The sugar content is high and he needs to try other foods too. We also suggest that you avoid straw-berries and citrus fruits in his first year as they are common allergens.

Don't forget to include a wide variety of vegetables in the foods you offer your baby. Raw vegetables can easily be cut into finger-size portions, but you must wash them first. Soak them in water and vinegar, rinse well and peel them if the skin is tough. This is especially impor-tant if they are not organically grown. Children love the crunchy quality of raw vegetables, but always make sure your child is supervised while eating things like carrot or celery and that he sits quietly. It's unlikely, but if a piece of food should go down the wrong way, put your child over your knee so that his head is lower than his chest and give him four sharp blows just between his shoulder blades. Don't attempt to do this while he is sitting upright, as the food may become more securely lodged.

You can vary the taste and texture of vegetables by stir-frying them with a little olive oil and garlic, or by adding a dash of tamari sauce or vinaigrette (use cold-pressed olive oil and apple cider vinegar). It's probably a good idea to leave the introduction of the nightshade family (potatoes, capsicums, eggplant and tomatoes) until he's 12 months old, and to avoid whole nuts until he's 2, since they can present a choking hazard.

Introduce meat by giving your baby a chop or chicken drumstick to suck. Later, when he's at least a year old, you can give him a thin strip of meat to chew; your dog can always deal with the remains.

Fish means fresh fish, not the fingers that masquerade under the title of fish—they contain all sorts of chemicals and preservatives (and precious little fish). Deep-sea fish is the least polluted and therefore the best choice for your baby. Shellfish should be avoided until your baby reaches 24 months since it is a common allergen.

Yoghurt goes well with sweet or savoury things and is a good source of protein and calcium. Since it is pre-digested it is unlikely to cause the gastrointestinal problems in an immature gut that are common with other dairy products. Make sure that it is cultured and that it contains lactobacillus, but is free of sugar and flavourings or other additives. Yoghurt helps to maintain healthy levels of bacteria in the gut and can reduce the chance of allergies.

Grains that you can try after 6 months include rice, buckwheat, millet, quinoa and couscous, but make sure that they are very well cooked to aid digestion. Leave the introduction of the 'big grasses'— wheat, rye, barley and oats—until your baby is at least 12 months old.

Eggs, though a good source of protein, are a very common allergen. The white is the main cause of the problem, so you can give your baby yolk, but only if it's mixed with other foods, and only after he is at least 6 months of age. Eggwhite may be introduced later, with caution, and must always be cooked.

Remember that your baby has been getting most, if not all, of his fluids from your milk. He will need to learn to drink from a bottle, or a cup, and will require plenty of purified water. Don't give him lots of fluids just before or during a meal, as this will fill him up and dilute the digestive juices in his stomach.

If at any time you have to resort to using pre-prepared baby foods, choose those that are made from organically grown produce and guaranteed free from pesticides and other additives. Most commercial baby foods contain gluten, cow's milk, sugars and additives such as fillers, as well as genetically engineered products.

Introduce one food at a time

Once your baby starts to reach for solid food, try to restrict him to one new food at a time and limit the introduction of a new food to once every two or three days (and never when he is sick). In this way you can watch carefully for any symptoms that might indicate he is not yet ready for that particular food. The things to watch for include gastrointestinal upsets (diarrhoea or constipation), nappy rash, sneezing, coughing, runny nose, ear infections, skin rashes, behaviour changes, changed sleep patterns, colic or excessive crying. A sudden onset of any of these (or other) conditions may indicate that your baby is allergic or intolerant to the new food (see more below).

Avoid the troublesome food for the time being and try it again in a month or two when his digestive system has matured a little more. Don't force him under any circumstances to eat a food that seems to disagree with him, simply because you think it's good for him. If he is happy to try most new tastes and flavours but exhibits a definite distaste for a particular food, respect his body's innate wisdom. He may know something about his ability to digest it that you don't!

A varied menu

Once your baby's eating a wide variety of nutritious foods, small frequent snacks throughout the day may be more appropriate for him than three large meals. The snacks don't need to be specially prepared. Use and modify what you're eating yourself but don't offer the same things day after day. Rotate menus so that your baby receives the widest possible variety of foods. Along with the too early introduction of solids, the frequency of exposure has a great deal to do with the development of allergy or intolerance (see more on this below).

Avoid refined sugars

It goes without saying that good nutrition is important for your growing baby, and good nutrition for his brain, which continues to develop at a very rapid rate for the first three years of his life, is absolutely vital. The brain, which controls mood, mind, memory and behaviour, depends on a stable supply of glucose to fuel all of its processes. In other words, the energy for all brain functions, which also include the control of hormones, regulation of breathing rate, control of motor activity and sense perception is supplied by a simple sugar.

However, not one molecule of refined sugar is needed by the brain— or by any other part of the body—to fuel any of its processes. Despite the catchy slogan of the sugar industry— 'It's a natural part of life'—that is one thing that sugar most definitely is not. In fact, the consumption of refined sugar which approaches 50 kilos per person per year is the most profound dietary change mankind has ever experienced. That amounts to more than half a cup of refined sugar every day; to get that amount of sugar from unrefined sources you would need to eat about 1 kilo of sugar beet or consume several metres of sugar cane.

Choose complex carbohydrates

So how are those needs for glucose to be fulfilled? Complex carbo-hydrates are found in wholegrains such as rice, buckwheat, quinoa, oats, barley and wheat, in legumes such as lentils and chickpeas, in varieties of beans and in fruit and vegetables. They are composed of sugar molecules linked together. Some of these long chains of sugar molecules are indigestible and form the fibre in food; others are broken down by the body to form simple sugars such as glucose. The important point about the digestion of complex carbohydrates is that they are broken down to glucose molecules over a period of hours. In other words, glucose is supplied to the brain at a steady rate and all the functions that the brain controls proceed uniformly and appropriately.

Refined sugar leads to blood sugar swings

Something different happens with a high intake of refined sugar, which you can think of as pre-digested complex carbohydrates. Refined sugar is broken down to glucose in minutes, leading to high blood levels of glucose. The body reacts to these high glucose levels and secretes insulin. This takes the circulating glucose out of the bloodstream and stores it in the liver as glycogen (or later converts it to fat). This production of insulin causes the blood levels of glucose to fall below the normal, so you experience a swing from an excess of glucose to a deficit. When the brain receives too much or too little fuel, there is an alteration in its function. Babies and small children are particularly susceptible to fluctuating blood sugar levels since they often consume a relatively large amount of sugar for their small body weight. Though the consumption of refined sugars becomes more problematic when your child reaches toddler age, it's worthwhile understanding the negative effects it may have on your baby too.

What happens to your baby's brain in the hypo- or hyper-glycaemic state depends to a large extent on individual biochemistry and personality type. He may be irritable or cranky, fretful, anxious, whingeing or sleepy. An older child may become uncontrollable, unable to stop himself, deaf to parental pleas and disciplinary action. He may be unable to concentrate fully. His co-ordination may be affected. He may become clumsy or unable to complete normally achievable tasks. Some effects will be unmistakable while others will be subtle. They may simply be dismissed as carelessness or boredom; you might perhaps think that is the way babies or small children are meant to be.

But no matter what the symptoms, your child will respond to low sugar levels with a demand for what is lacking. He will want another sugary snack knowing that it makes him feel better and the cycle will repeat itself. Ingestion of large quantities of pure apple juice, which contains the natural sugars of tens of apples, may produce similar symptoms.

The same effects can be observed when your baby or child goes too long without food, so frequent snacks can be more helpful than infrequent, large meals. As protein takes longer to digest, it can keep blood sugar levels stable for longer than other foods.

Sugar leads to long-term health problems

The short-term implications of eating refined sugars are obvious. Further down the track, constant high circulating levels of insulin contribute to fatigue, to obesity and to a host of chronic degenerative conditions. Too much sugar also has a depressant effect on the immune system and is responsible for increasing cholesterol levels and platelet stickiness. Also, nutrients including B-complex vitamins and trace minerals such as zinc, magnesium and chromium are needed for the metabolism of sugar and starch. However, these are lost during the refining processes, so eating a diet containing a high proportion of sugary products can lead to a deficiency in many essential nutrients. And in the long term this constant stress on the pancreas can trigger adult onset diabetes when, due to a lifetime of overuse, the production of insulin ceases altogether. Unfortunately, due to our society's love affair with sugar, the incidence of diabetes is growing rapidly and becoming one of the major threats to health and life-expectancy.

Do not be tempted to sweeten foods for your baby to make them more palatable. Your strength now will stand you in good stead later when he is starting preschool and is exposed to advertising and the pressure of his peer group, and begins to demand inappropriate food and drink. If you've already established good eating habits it will be so much easier to explain to your child why you limit his access to refined and processed products. We'll look very closely at optimal nutrition for preschool children (and older) in our next book, *The Natural Way to Raise a Better Baby* but meanwhile you can be sure it's never too early to start good habits and never too late for you to set a good example. If you and your partner eat well, your child will follow. Chapter 5 sets out our recommendations for optimum nutrition—both you and your child will benefit if you live by its advice.

WEANING YOUR TODDLER

Avoid cow's milk

Humans are the only creatures on earth that regularly drink the milk designed for another species. So weaning your older child doesn't mean replacing breast milk with cow's milk. As we have seen above, it is the most common allergen, and calcium, iron and other nutrients are poorly absorbed from cow's milk. Two-thirds of the world's population cannot tolerate milk, butter or cheese and get their calcium requirements from other sources. These include cultured yoghurt (which is tolerated better than other dairy products by most people as it is pre-digested by the bacteria in the culture), tahini paste, green leafy vegetables and fish with edible bones such as salmon and sardines. Remember, too that other minerals such as magnesium and zinc are important for the development of strong bones and teeth. Cow's milk clogs the arteries of babies and young children and will reduce your child's appetite for more nourishing foods. Goat's milk is a possible alternative if you simply must give your child a milk drink.

Limit soy consumption

Unfortunately soy milk is not really an alternative drink for your toddler either. With a huge increase in the consumption of soy milk over the last twenty years, we are now seeing an increase in the number of children who are allergic to soy. As we have seen, soy can also interfere with the formation of hormone receptor sites and can block the absorption of proteins and essential minerals.

As well, soy is not a primary protein and needs to be combined with other plant protein to provide all the essential amino acids. Some brands may be high in sugars, may have a high aluminium content, which is an extra burden for immature kidneys, and may contain genetically modified beans. Even those brands that state 'No genetically engineered beans' may contain a food additive that has been manufactured from a genetically engineered product.

Limit fruit juice consumption

Over the last 25 years in the West the consumption of fruit juice has increased from about 40 mL per capita to 270 mL a day. Fruit juices contain the sugar of tens of apples, oranges, pears or other fruit, and their consumption has been linked to dental decay and chronic non-specific diarrhoea (especially if sorbitol is present). Juice dilutes the acid in the stomach and reduces the absorption of nutrients, and since the child's stomach is very small, juice may also reduce his appetite for food. Children drinking more than 360 mL of juice per day have been shown to suffer from stunted growth and obesity.

Water is the answer

If you're wondering what on earth you're going to give your child to drink, rest assured that purified water is still impossible to beat as a thirst quencher. Fruit smoothies made with an overripe banana, some unsweetened yoghurt and water can make a change from what comes out of the tap. You can vary the smoothie flavour by using a different variety of fruit.

FOOD ALLERGIES AND INTOLERANCES

Sometimes, as we've already discussed, a fully breastfed child can react inappropriately to a food that you eat. Alternatively, your child may display telltale allergic symptoms when you introduce solid food. If you've read all of our previous books and followed our recommendations, then your chances of having a child suffering from food allergy or intolerance is very slight. But you should be aware that a significant number of physical, mental and emotional conditions are due to inappropriate reactions to specific foods. The most common allergens include cow's milk and cheese, wheat, gluten-containing grains (such as rye, oats and corn), eggs, chicken, yeast, pork, peanuts and citrus fruits.

Because of your child's immaturity and his small physical size, and because his brain is still developing, he is especially sensitive to offending compounds. The symptoms that he exhibits may be quite different from those exhibited by an adult reacting to the same substances. Unfortunately, it's possible for your child to suffer from allergy or intolerance even when he's breastfed and eating a really excellent diet.

Symptoms of allergy and intolerance

The symptoms that an allergic or intolerant child might display are extremely varied. We've already mentioned colic and prolonged crying, nappy rash, eczema, diarrhoea, constipation, colds and runny noses, middle ear infections and sleep disturbances. To complicate matters, the way in which an allergy or intolerance manifests may change as your child matures. For example, your toddler may be prone to tantrums or he may run around in a wild, haphazard fashion, touching everything in sight with absolutely no sense of danger. He might suffer from nightmares. As he grows older he may have frequent headaches or stomach-aches, unexplained joint and muscle pain, or he may continue to wet the bed. He may develop glue ear or suffer from asthma. Many of the symptoms of allergy or intolerance are neurological—your child may be clumsy, he may have difficulty completing a task, trouble with reading or with mathematical calculations and he might be disruptive in class or at home.

Sadly, lots of these health and behaviour patterns are dismissed as simply a function of being a baby or child. Many parents are unaware of their children's allergies and sensitivities, and as the adverse response becomes chronic, it's accepted as 'just the way things are'. If you suspect that allergy or intolerance is a problem, then it's worth considering some of the approaches and diagnostic methods that we have outlined in Chapter 10, or consulting a natural health practitioner who specialises in allergy detection. A practitioner may be able to help you devise a realistic dietary plan if you are having difficulty sorting one out yourself, but eating according to our recommendations and avoiding prolonged or frequent contact with allergens will make a considerable difference. Of course a strong immune system is your child's best defence against allergy, and good nutrition is an essential precursor to this, but ironically this is a chicken-and-egg situation, so the allergy must be effectively dealt with first.

Other factors implicated in allergy

You might notice that your baby or child does not always react adversely to a problem food. The display of symptoms can depend on the total load of stressors that are present at any one time. Some of the other factors that might contribute to allergy or intolerance include:

- pollutants in unpurified water (pesticides, flocculants)
- additives in food (preservatives, colourings)
- compromised nutritional status (especially zinc deficiency)
- stress (teething, weaning)
- airborne pollutants (low cloud cover, high pollen levels, strong winds blowing off the land, local agricultural spraying)

- high body burden of toxic metals (especially lead, but also copper, aluminium, cadmium and mercury—see Chapter 6)
- other subtle influences (e.g. fluorescent lights, television, noise, colour)

To help you distinguish between the influence of these factors and a food allergy, it's helpful to keep a food diary. In this you can record the foods eaten by your child in the 6,12 and 24 hours before any reaction or behaviour which you consider may have been triggered by allergy. On reviewing the patterns that emerge, you may well find that one or more specific foods crop up over and over again.

BREASTFED BABIES ARE SMALLER, BUT HEALTHIER

It's worthwhile knowing that if you leave the introduction of solids until well into the second half of your breastfed baby's first year, he'll be smaller than a bottle-fed baby of the same age and also smaller than a baby who's had solids from an early age. And, if you've followed our dietary recommendations all through your pregnancy and while you've been breastfeeding, you might find he's smaller than the breastfed baby of a woman eating a typical Western diet that is high in refined carbohydrates, sugar and fat. However, this does not mean he will grow into a smaller child or adult, and your smaller, fully breastfed baby is not necessarily lighter than his bottle-fed counterparts. His bones are denser and he has a higher proportion of lean muscle, which means he may well be heavier. Remember, too, that fat cells are laid down in infancy, and large, chubby babies may be in for a lifelong battle with excess weight. So all in all, if you keep breastfeeding and delay introducing solids a little, your baby will be optimally healthy, but you'll have to put up with a fair bit of societal pressure.

It might help you to feel justified in your stance if we quote the new resolution of the World Health Organisation—issued in May 2001, which urges Member States to:

> . . . support exclusive breastfeeding for six months as a global public health recommendation taking into account the findings of the WHO Expert Technical Consultation on optimal duration of exclusive breastfeeding and to provide safe and appropriate complementary foods, with continued breastfeeding for up to two years or beyond . . .

Sexuality and contraception during breastfeeding

After the birth of your baby, especially if it's your first, your relationship with your partner will change in many ways, and this may include the way you relate sexually.

WHAT HAPPENED TO SEX?

Many women feel relatively sexually uninterested after childbirth and during breastfeeding. So if this is happening to you, you're not alone or being overreactive. It's quite normal and natural to feel this way, and all part of Mother Nature's plan to help space your children in the most effective and healthy manner. Don't worry about it! The feeling is not only normal, and a natural way to achieve birth control, but it will pass.

Indeed studies show a wide variation of sexual behaviour among women at this time. This may help to reassure you that your response—whatever it may be—isn't unusual. Masters and Johnson found that the time taken to return to pre-pregnancy levels of sexual activity varied from a few weeks to three months or more. Other studies show that some women have still not resumed sexual intercourse after a year. Only 35–50 per cent of women are sexually active within six weeks, and 88 per cent at 12 weeks. Every woman is different and no response is better than another. You'll need to take it at your own pace.

In fact, in some cultures post-childbirth sexual abstinence is compulsory, and it is considered bad form for children to be born very close together. For example, in Sierra Leone sexual abstinence lasts for a full year after birth; in some Pacific Island cultures it lasts for two. While we don't want you to feel that there's necessarily a need for any period of sexual inactivity, we also want you to feel that there are recognised traditions and sound reasons for taking your time and waiting until you feel comfortable.

Although some women experience a highly charged vitality, even in the first few days after birth, and find their sexual energy also heightened, there are many reasons why you may be less sexually motivated than before. You need to explore these underlying conditions and do what's best for you (and your partner). The factors involved include hormonal changes, your new role as a mother (and your joint role as parents), your levels of energy, your emotional state, physical problems resulting from childbirth, your new body image, your possible fear of another pregnancy and your partner's attitude to it all. As well as learning to let your body and libido recover at their own rate, there's a lot that can be done to remedy many of these problems.

Your hormones affect your libido

While you're breastfeeding, raised levels of prolactin are produced by your pituitary gland. This is the hormone that controls lactation and, as we saw in Chapter 2, it also has a sedative effect. Another result of increased prolactin production is that ovulation is delayed (we'll look at this again when we discuss how it affects fertility). In the absence of an ovulation cycle, normal ovarian hormones such as oestrogen won't peak once a month to trigger the release of an egg, and this affects your sexual motivation.

The majority of women feel most highly sexual when they are fertile, at ovulation. (Nature has a benign conspiracy with our bodies to have us reproduce as often as possible.) We have also observed that women who are aware of their lunar cycle and its effects on their fertility (more of this towards the end of this chapter) find that their sexuality is heightened when they are at their 'lunar peak'; that is, at the time when their fertility is increased due to this biorhythm. So, in the absence of fertility and ovulation, sexual desire is lowered, as nature has no pay-off in terms of reproduction.

In Chapter 2 we also looked at how oxytocin, the hormone respon-sible for the let-down reflex, is the same hormone that is released at orgasm, and how this may also affect your attitude to sex. It may make you less likely to look for sexual satisfaction with your partner, or it may increase your sexuality and act as an aphrodisiac.

Your new role as a mother

Part of the delight you take in your new baby will be sensual. The skin-to-skin contact, so vital for him, is also exquisitely pleasurable for you. This, coupled with the intense feelings of love you feel, will probably mean that you are emotionally and physically focused on your child, and on your breastfeeding relationship. This doesn't mean that you care less for your partner, simply that you may be distracted by your new experiences. Although this is a natural survival mechanism to protect and nurture your tiny baby, your partner may need some reassurance that he's still important to you.

For some women, this physical focus on their baby is almost over-whelming, and they feel that any further tactile or sensual experience, after the 20 hours a day spent with their baby, is just sensory overload. If you're feeling like this, you may crave time on your own without having to 'give out' to anyone else, and time to have your body to yourself. You'll need to explain this need to your family so they won't feel rejected.

However, few modern mothers are able to ignore the demands of daily life for long, and your partner, and any older children, have legiti-mate claims to your care and attention. Conversation about nappies and feeding schedules may not be what they require, and you may need to make an effort to switch your attention to subjects that aren't related to matters infantile. On the other hand, you may well find yourself craving adult and intellectual conversation, even if you don't yet feel like sexual activity.

It's a common joke that birth control in the postnatal period is mostly achieved through 'baby interruptus'. You may be distracted during the time you spend with your partner because a large part of your attention is focused on listening for your baby, fearing that he may wake up. In fact, many babies seem to have an internal alarm that rings just as you and your partner are finally making some headway in the romantic stakes. The best way round this is to keep your baby in (or at least near) the bed with you. In this way he will sense that you are close and stay peacefully asleep. Even if he does wake, you can tend to him without too much disturbance.

You may be tired or depressed

However well you manage your night-time feeds, and even if your baby is free from conditions such as colic (which can disturb your nights), you may still find at the end of the day, or at any time when you can relax, that all you want to do is sleep, and that sex is the furthest thing from your mind. Obviously the best plan is to sleep when your baby does, but this may not leave much room (or desire) for sexual activity. It may also mean that your partner's and your timetables don't synchronise, as he may not be able, or want, to adapt his to yours, and you may be waking and sleeping at different times. If you feel like ships passing in the night, make 'appointments' to at least meet and talk, and arrange to set aside special times to get together.

Fatigue is a real problem for many new mothers, and certainly doesn't predispose you to sexual activity. If you are flexible with your sleep patterns, this will help, but a lot will also depend on your nutritional status. It'll be easier if you've attended to this before the birth, or, even better, before the conception (see our previous books), but you can still improve your energy levels considerably by attending to the ideas in Chapter 5; that is, eating well and supplementing sensibly.

Good nutrition (especially adequate zinc status) is also a prerequisite if you want to avoid postnatal depression. Poor nutritional status and sleep deprivation are perhaps the two main contributing factors to this condition. In our previous book, *Healthy Body, Better Birthing*, you'll find lots of advice for self-help and natural remedies, but if depression persists you should seek professional help. Postnatal depression can be very debilitating, and will certainly prevent your libido returning at its natural rate.

Physical recovery from childbirth

Depending on your experience of childbirth, for a while afterwards you may well feel that your genital area could do with a rest. Your perineum may be quite bruised, or you may have had stitches after a tear or an episiotomy. You'll be less likely to have experienced these—and even if you have, recovery will be much faster—if you've attended to your nutrition (especially your zinc levels) pre and postnatally.

Full details of remedies for recovery can be found in *Healthy Body, Better Birthing*, but *Arnica* or *Witch Hazel* ointments used topically (though not on broken skin) can be very helpful for bruising, and *Arnica* can also be taken internally as a homoeopathic remedy. You can try sitz-baths with essential oils such as *Lavender* or the herbs *Calendula* and *Comfrey* to aid healing of tears or cuts. Poultices or compresses made with these essential oils and herbs can also help. *St John's Wort (Hypericum)* oil is particularly helpful to heal any damaged nerve endings. Obviously, even if you felt like it, penetrative sexual activity should not be resumed until all stitches are removed and any cuts or tears are healed. The bleeding and discharge (called lochia) that normally last between 2–4 weeks after childbirth are quite normal, and should not prevent sexual activity if you feel inclined.

You may feel that your vagina has changed a lot and that your vaginal muscles are very slack. Just as the practice of pelvic floor exercises prenatally will help prevent this problem, so they can now help to resolve it (see Chapter 7 for details). Good nutrition can help too. Eat foods rich in calcium and magnesium (almond and brazil nuts make great snacks) and supplement with these nutrients too, since they are essential for muscle contraction.

The low levels of oestrogen that you experience when you're not ovulating (or menstruating) not only reduce your libido, but can contribute to vaginal dryness, which doesn't make sex any more attractive. Also, the glands producing lubrication may not be working well at first, so you may need to use lots of lubrication when you do resume intercourse. You'll find that plenty of foreplay will help you to secrete more easily, especially if it includes relaxing and comforting activities like massage and stroking.

'My breasts aren't mine anymore'

You may feel that your breasts are not yours anymore, and that they have been taken over by your baby. It may be difficult to relate to them as a sexual organ while they are a source of nourishment for your child. Of course sex and reproduction are all part of the same cycle, and if you can truly understand or intuitively feel that, it may make it easier to resolve any conflicting feelings you have. (Your partner may need to try to do this too!)

If you have problems such as cracked nipples, engorgement or mastitis, the last thing you'll want is anyone touching your breasts, and of course this will also affect your breastfeeding (see Chapter 10 for some helpful natural remedies).

Some women find it difficult to relate to their 'new' breasts, which may be much larger and fuller than they were before. Often this process has been happening all through pregnancy, and you'll have had time to adapt. In fact you may well be very pleased with your new figure and you (and your partner) may find it quite a turn-on. However, leaking breasts certainly present a challenge, especially as this can be triggered by sexual arousal. This is where humour and a few well-placed pads and towels can save the day. Your partner may even develop a taste for breast milk.

Body image may be a problem

You may feel, after childbirth, that your body looks and feels unattractive, and isn't sexy anymore. This is partly to do with your own expectations of what makes someone sexually attractive, and what you feel your partner's attitude may be. It may also involve your partner's expressed or apparent feelings on the matter.

Many women regain their figure easily and fast. But it's natural to be different from your pre-pregnant state, and one of those differences may be increased weight. Now is not a good time for dieting, though if you eat and exercise as we've suggested, you may find that the kilos drop off quite quickly. If not, you're going to need to make friends with your new body and learn to appreciate your voluptuous curves and more rounded shape in order to reclaim your sexuality. Acceptance will come more easily if you are able to see how motherhood is part of sexuality, and also if you had a positive attitude to your pregnancy and birth. If you had a good birth and supportive carers this will help too.

It's difficult to persuade anyone that stretch marks and flabby tummies are sexually attractive, but if you have these you should wear them with pride as a badge of your motherhood. If you achieved good nutrition (especially adequate zinc levels) during and before pregnancy, this will have helped to prevent stretch marks, and good muscle tone can be achieved through both nutrition and exercise.

Fear of another pregnancy

Even if you haven't resumed ovulating or menstruating yet, and are presently unable to conceive, your fear of another pregnancy coming too soon could well inhibit your sexual response. In order to allay these fears, you need to have confidence in your contraception, and we hope that the information contained later in this chapter will enable you to feel that you have this under control and that you can relax and focus on regaining intimacy with your partner.

Your partner's attitude

Your partner may also be experiencing problems, which may leave him unable to offer you the support you need to resolve yours. His libido may have received a jolt too, which could compound your difficulties. Some men who attend the birth of their child find they are strongly affected by the experience. It arouses in them a desire to protect their spouse, and they may be afraid of causing hurt. Alternatively they may have reacted negatively to the experience, and become turned off by their perception of the female genitalia as traumatised and unattractive. Other men find it difficult to relate to their partner as both mother and lover, and they may need to learn how to see both of these roles as manifestations of womanhood.

Another problem can arise if your partner feels left out of the close relationship developing between you and your baby. Some men become quite jealous, resentful of the time you spend with your child and impatient with your lack of energy for other concerns (notably him). He may feel that your baby has 'stolen' your body, and that your breasts, which were once there for him, have been usurped by a hungry infant. He may also feel overwhelmed by their new size and the milk that spurts everywhere.

You'll need to talk each other's feelings through, and both of you will need to be patient. What's most important is that you communicate your feelings, offer mutual support, and agree on how and when you'll resume sexual activity. If you don't, you could end up having a bad sexual experience, alienating each other, and affecting your sex life for a lot longer than necessary.

HOW AND WHEN TO RESUME SEX

When you resume sex is really up to the two of you and how you feel (as we've outlined above). As for how, we can give you a few ideas.

Start gently. There are many ways you can express yourselves sexually and sensually which don't have to lead to intercourse. Sheila Kitzinger recommends that the first few sexual encounters should not include penetration. Instead you could caress each other with your hands or engage in oral sex.

When you do resume penetration, you'll need lots of lubrication and foreplay. Experiment with position. Some counsellors advise avoiding the missionary position, as this presses on the rear wall of the vagina, which may be sore. But not everyone is sore in the same spot, so gently try out some different angles to see which is most comfortable for you. And relax! Worrying won't change anything except by making things worse; if you let it all unfold naturally, you can be confident you'll be a fully functional sexual being again in good time.

BREASTFEEDING: NATURE'S WAY OF SPACING CHILDREN

It is commonly observed that second and subsequent children are frequently not as healthy as first children, and studies confirm that an interval of approximately two years between conceptions and births is optimal. This may well underlie some of the traditional customs of enforced sexual abstinence we spoke of earlier. The mother needs time to recover, both physically and emotionally, from the nutritional and other demands made upon her. Her next child's health will suffer if this recovery is not complete before her next conception. With adequate spacing between births, the older child will benefit from being the sole recipient of her attention and her breast milk.

However, full abstinence is not the only way to achieve optimal child spacing. Breastfeeding provides its own considerable protection against conception. Nature steps in once again, her grand design ensuring a protracted period of infertility after childbirth due to lactational amenorrhoea (the absence of periods due to breastfeeding).

Pre-twentieth century records from communities around the world where breast milk was the primary source of food for babies up to eighteen months of age, show that the average time between births was approximately two years. Some studies assess the risk of conception in the first six months after a birth for a woman who is fully and frequently breastfeeding as about 1 per cent: a better rate than that offered by the mini-pill. This low rate is dependent on a woman allowing her baby to suckle whenever he wants to (sometimes called 'ecological breastfeeding'). Fully breastfeeding also means there are no complementary bottles of formula, the breast is used as a pacifier, the baby feeds during the night and has not been introduced to solids. If you wish to fully experience the contraceptive effect of breastfeeding you *must* follow these guidelines. You can then be reasonably confident of remaining infertile for the first 10 or even 12 weeks after childbirth so long as you have experienced no bleeding since the end of the blood-stained discharge (called lochia) that follows the birth. Compare this with a woman who is not breastfeeding who can only confidently consider herself infertile for the first 2–3 weeks and will probably have a period within 6–12 weeks.

However, the pattern of lactational amenorrhoea is different in individual instances, though most women find that the length of time before their first bleed tends to be similar after each birth. Breastfeeding patterns can be vulnerable to external influences, especially with our modern lifestyles and, as we shall see, lactation is not the only factor influencing the return of fertility. Because of this, breastfeeding is not a foolproof method of contraception and further studies have shown that between 10 and 20 per cent of breastfeeding women ovulate, and could conceive, within 12 weeks of giving birth.

These women may well be those in our Western culture who go back to work and use all manner of tricks to get their babies to sleep through the night. However, in another study in Western Samoa, where the women fully breastfeed their babies for up to three years, most women resumed menstruation after one month and frequently had two babies within the same year. So you can see how the success of the contraceptive effect can vary, and depend on the circumstances. Luckily there are other natural methods available which will not harm the health of you or your baby, which can support the contraceptive effect of breastfeeding, and which allow you to take advantage of this often quite lengthy infertile time, when the use of continuous chemical or mechanical birth control is quite unnecessary. We will look at these other natural methods—mucus checking, temperature reading and plotting your 'lunar' cycle—later in the chapter. But first, let's look at how the contraceptive effect of breastfeeding is achieved.

Breastfeeding delays ovulation

Prolactin, a pituitary hormone present in high levels during lactation, delays ovulation in most women through its sterilising action on the ovaries. If you fully breastfeed during the first six months, and then partially breastfeed, but use the breast as a pacifier (especially at night), you are unlikely to ovulate before 9–12 months, even though you may bleed. (It will be an anovular cycle; that is, one with no ovulation.) Although we have known of a few conceptions occurring within three weeks of birth and are therefore cautious about giving the following advice, you can generally consider yourself safe from conception for the first 10 weeks after birth, and at low risk for the first 16 if you are allowing your baby to feed on demand. The risk then starts to increase, with a 6–9 per cent chance of conception occurring before your first menstruation. This is because your first ovulation may precede your first menstrual period, especially if your periods resume later than nine months postpartum.

So you can see it's very important for you to be aware of the signs that can tell you of an imminent ovulation. The observance of these signs forms the basis of the natural methods of fertility management—mucus checking and temperature reading—that you can use to supplement the contraceptive effects of breastfeeding.

Other factors affecting the return of fertility

The duration of your postpartum infertility will be affected by a number of other factors, as well as the frequency of your baby's feeds. One of these factors is stress. However, unlike the pre-pregnant situation, stress is likely to precipitate, not delay, ovulation if you are breastfeeding. This is because its effect on prolactin levels is different when you are lactating, reducing its production, diminishing your ability to feed and increasing the chances of ovulation.

Frequency of sexual activity will also influence the rate at which your fertility is restored. Sexuality and fertility are linked, and if you engage in a full and active sex life during breastfeeding, this will hasten the return of your menstrual cycle.

As we've already seen, sexuality may well be subdued during breast-feeding, and this may also be part of nature's way of spacing your children. The lack of ovulation and low hormone levels lead to a reduction in libido, which leads to less sexual activity, which, in turn, leads to a lack of ovulation. Neat, isn't it? However, those of you who manage to outwit nature and remain sexually active will need to be careful with your contraception.

So to summarise, the factors involved in restoring your fertility include:

- less sucking
- using a dummy instead of the breast
- cutting out night feeds
- introducing solids
- introducing complementary formula bottles
- weaning
- stress
- frequent sexual activity

Francesca has developed a rule which may make all this easier to remember. It's called Francesca's Five Fs Rule and it goes like this: The less you Feed, and the more you Fuss or Frolic, the Faster your Fertility will return.

Be warned, however, that there are always occasional exceptions to these rules, and it may be wise to start observing the signs of returning fertility and using the back-up forms of natural contraception that we outline below from the very beginning. First, let's look at why some other popular methods of contraception may not be suitable at this time.

CONVENTIONAL CONTRACEPTION DURING BREASTFEEDING

Of course, the only 100 per cent effective form of contraception is abstinence (and by that we mean no genital contact, as even external contact without penetration has a slight chance of causing a conception). Despite our earlier thoughts on why your sex drive may be somewhat reduced, we're not really recommending this for any but the most determined couples! However, it may be a realistic option if you only need to abstain at those times when you may be able to conceive. This will depend on learning to tell confidently when you are fertile and when you are not (see below).

Some women are prescribed the mini-pill after they've given birth, but we'll look at why the breastfeeding period is a totally inappropriate time to be using chemical means of contraception. An IUD may be recommended for some women, and although its insertion is easier after childbirth, risks such as pelvic inflammatory disease and side effects such as increased bleeding and pain at menstruation have justifiably made this an increasingly unpopular option.

Barrier methods such as condoms and diaphragms present few, if any, health concerns, though they may well contribute to your disinclination to have intercourse. They are extremely reliable, if used correctly, and can be combined with the methods we'll describe which enable you to tell when you're fertile, thus reducing the number of occasions on which they're required.

If you choose to use a diaphragm, it's important that you are refitted at your first postnatal check-up, about six weeks after the birth, as you will probably need a larger size than you did before pregnancy. You may also need to check the size again about six months later. Because you may be experiencing some vaginal dryness, condoms will need to be well lubricated—you may find that the lubricant with which they're already impregnated is not sufficient.

In Francesca's book *Natural Fertility*, you can find out more about the disadvantages, advantages and guidelines associated with these and other methods of contraception. However, because it is so often prescribed during breastfeeding, we want to summarise here some of our concerns about the use of the mini-pill.

Oral contraceptives are not the answer

The artificial hormones in the oral contraceptive pill rely on several effects to prevent contraception. The combination pill, which contains both oestrogen and progesterone, acts in three ways:

- sterilisation—inhibiting ovarian activity
- abortion—altering the womb's lining to prevent implantation
- contraception—making the mucus in the cervix hostile to sperm

The mini-pill contains only progesterone. It does not inhibit ovulation, relying on the second and third actions only for its contraceptive effect. Because oestrogen interferes with your metabolism and could have an inhibiting effect on lactation, the combination pill is unlikely to be prescribed. However, the progesterone in the commonly prescribed mini-pill is secreted in your breast milk, and may also have several adverse effects including the following.

- It changes the taste of the milk, which can affect feeding.
- It affects the nutritional content of your milk (see below).
- It is known to act on the hypothalamus, and may have effects such as masculinisation of a female infant, who is forming her hormone receptor sites soon after birth.
- The ingestion of chemical hormones is inappropriate for babies of either sex during this critical developmental period (this is another compelling reason to also avoid the synthetic oestrogen of the combination pill, especially if you have a male baby).
- It may contribute to neonatal jaundice.

It is also of concern that the mini-pill needs to be taken at approximately the same time of day to be effective. This can be tricky if your routine is interrupted by an unpredictable baby. Because of this, the effective rate of contraception may not be acceptable. If conception does occur while you are taking the mini-pill, there is an increased risk of ectopic pregnancy. This is because you may still ovulate, but the passage of the egg or sperm through the Fallopian tubes may be affected.

Although there are clear contraindications for mini-pill use, many prescriptions are given without a sufficiently thorough investigation of your personal health history. This is particularly important at this time as, during pregnancy and postnatally, you may have suffered from some health conditions with which you had no previous problems. For a full list refer to *Natural Fertility* but, in summary, it's particularly important to avoid any sort of pill use if you have a personal or family history of:

- cardiovascular disease (including hypertension)
- diabetes
- liver, gall bladder or kidney disease
- irregularities of menstruation
- reproductive or breast cancer, cysts or tumours
- epilepsy or multiple sclerosis
- depression (including postnatal depression)
- migraines or recurrent headache
- candida (vaginal or systemic)
- allergy or dysfunction of the immune system

There are many reasons why you should not conceive while taking, or soon after ceasing to take, oral contraception, including a higher incidence of stillbirths, miscarriages and congenital abnormalities. Many of these problems may be attributable to the adverse effect on your nutritional status. This is one of the main reasons we suggest that you should avoid it while you are breastfeeding, as it also affects the nutritional content of your milk. This is the last thing you need at a time when your baby's physical and mental growth is proceeding exponentially. Here is a list of nutrients and other factors that are affected in a woman using oral contraception (for more details see *Natural Fertility*):

- vitamin A
- vitamin B1
- vitamin B2
- vitamin B6
- vitamin B12
- folic acid
- biotin
- vitamin C
- bioflavonoids
- vitamin E
- vitamin K
- iron
- calcium
- magnesium
- potassium
- selenium
- copper
- zinc
- prostaglandins
- blood lipids

It has also been shown that the protein quality of your milk is affected if you take the mini-pill, as are the levels of fats. If you started at the beginning of this book and read Chapter 5 before this one, then you'll know why we're concerned.

HOW TO USE NATURAL BIRTH CONTROL WHEN YOU ARE BREASTFEEDING

If, like us, you are concerned about using the mini-pill while you are breastfeeding, and if you would like to restrict your use of abstinence or barrier methods to those times when you are likely to be at risk of conceiving, then it will be helpful to learn how to read the signs that nature has supplied to let you know when you are fertile.

There are two main observations which will be useful to you at this time. One is the change that occurs in the cervical mucus as you approach ovulation, and the other is the change in the body-at-rest temperature that occurs afterwards.

Cervical mucus and fertility

Change in the cervical mucus is the only observable symptom that precedes ovulation and therefore gives reliable warning of approaching fertility. Without this change, there is no fertility. Even if ovulation occurs, if there is no fertile mucus the situation is infertile, because sperm cannot stay alive.

So if you are aware of how your cervical mucus changes before you ovulate, you are always able to tell when your fertility is returning and you won't get caught out waiting for your first period (which, especially after the first nine months, will probably follow your first ovulation). You can therefore make love confidently during lactation, at your infertile times and, equally confidently, use barrier contraception or abstinence when your body is preparing to ovulate and until your fertile time has passed.

How does mucus checking work?

First you need to know that in favourable circumstances, sperm can live for up to three days. They have even been found alive after five, though this is extremely rare, and they are generally considered to be non-viable at this advanced age. Three days is usually considered to be their maximum viability. Sperm life reduces by one-third each day, and 16–18 hours is an average life span. The number of sperm (sperm count) also drops each day and, even in a favourable environment, falls below a viable level after three days.

However, acidity immobilises sperm, and vaginas are naturally acidic. Fertile mucus provides protection for the sperm from this acidity, it nourishes them and guides them up into the uterus. So you are therefore potentially fertile from the time this mucus first appears. Simply being aware of when you are ovulating may not be enough to protect you from conception, if you had intercourse up to three days previously. Mucus present at other times in the cycle (if any) is unable to provide the sperm with this protection and is, therefore, infertile.

The different types of mucus can all be identified under a microscope, but luckily the significant changes can also be differentiated by appearance and sensation. Gravity does the work for you and brings the mucus down to the mouth of the vagina, where changes in quality and quantity can be seen and felt.

A typical cycle progresses as follows.

- After bleeding there may be some dry days when there is no apparent mucus at all. (See below if your menstrual cycle has not yet resumed.) The mucus at this time is completely infertile and forms a plug across the cervix—this may come out as a blob of sticky mucus. Other women will experience small unchanging amounts of this thick, pasty, *infertile* mucus. This is called your Basic Infertile Pattern (BIP) which is essentially what you will experience when there is no ovarian hormonal activity.
- Then, as levels of oestrogen start to rise, you may start to feel the presence of some *possibly infertile* or *slightly fertile* mucus. This is usually a damp or sticky feeling.
- As oestrogen levels continue to rise, so does the water content in the mucus, which becomes wetter and more lubricative. This is the change to *fertile* mucus. It is also more profuse.
- As oestrogen levels peak, most women then experience the *spinnbarkeit* or 'spinn' mucus that resembles raw eggwhite and can be stretched between the fingers, while remaining wet to the touch. This mucus is *highly fertile*, and usually occurs just before ovulation.

- After ovulation there is a return, sometimes quite suddenly, to the thick, *infertile* mucus or to none at all (whichever constitutes your usual BIP).

It is these changes, which enable the sperm to survive and travel and which are your body's way of preparing for conception, that you can learn to recognise. They clearly define the approach of fertility, or lack of it. Every woman will experience some changes in her cervical mucus as she progresses through her hormonal cycle. All women do not experience all of the stages. They vary with the length of the cycle and the amount of mucus produced.

If you are using this method to avoid conception, three days must be allowed after the mucus has ceased to be fertile in order to be sure that ovulation is over. *Fertility starts as soon as the mucus changes as described above and lasts until three days after the last day of any type of fertile mucus. For contraceptive purposes you must avoid unprotected intercourse on these days.*

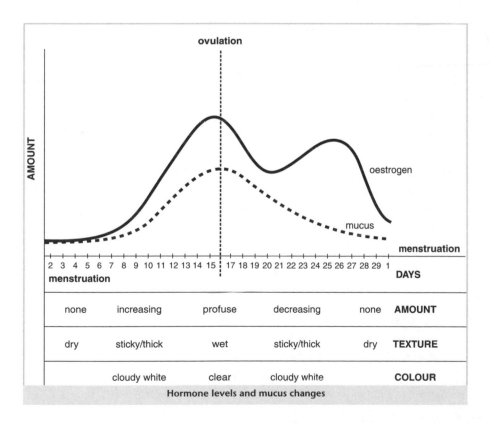

none	increasing	profuse	decreasing	none	AMOUNT
dry	sticky/thick	wet	sticky/thick	dry	TEXTURE
	cloudy white	clear	cloudy white		COLOUR

Hormone levels and mucus changes

How to use mucus observations while you are waiting for your cycle to return

Before your first ovulatory menstrual cycle after childbirth, you may not notice these changes at all or you may experience them in a random pattern. The important thing to identify is your Basic Infertile Pattern— the kind of mucus (if any) that you produce when nothing is happening as far as ovulation is concerned. You can recognise this because it will not change from day to day or over weeks. It may be that there is no mucus apparent at the mouth of the vagina, or that there are unchanging amounts of thick, pasty mucus just as you would expect once your cycle has resumed. However, during this postpartum period you may also find that you have unchanging amounts of wet mucus. Even though it is wet (which is normally considered fertile), if it is unchanging in quantity or quality over a period of time, you can consider this your Basic Infertile Pattern. If you have a day when all you have experienced is your Basic Inferntile Pattern you can consider that evening safe to have unprotected sex.

Often there will be a change in the Basic Infertile Pattern as your body goes through a series of 'I think I'll ovulate, I think I'll ovulate. No, I won't!' hiccoughs before eventually reasserting itself with 'Yes, I will!'. Although these are essentially false alarms, they must be taken seriously, as you won't know until later that no egg was released. It's therefore important to consider any change from the Basic Infertile Pattern as a possible preparation for an ovulation, and to take precautions or abstain until you have experienced three days of a return to the BIP.

If you used these methods before you conceived, you may now find that not only is your BIP different, but that the pattern of your cycle has also changed. Initially, you may have a longer pre-ovulatory phase and a shorter post-ovulatory phase—(your natural health practitioner can help if your cycle doesn't settle down). However, your mucus, if patiently watched, *will* warn you of your first ovulation. It's important to observe your mucus for changes as soon as you may be at risk of conception— we advise you start directly after childbirth, as soon as bleeding ceases.

How to check your mucus

Mucus is usually observed while seated on the toilet, before urinating, by collecting some from the vulval area (the mouth of the vagina), and assessing the texture and amount. These changes can then be charted, preferably with the help of a good teacher or teaching aid (see p. 174), and patterns will quickly become apparent once your cycle resumes. Although the observations will require some focused attention on your part before your cycle gets back into a regular pattern and for the first few cycles, your awareness of the mucus changes will soon become automatic, and you'll probably wonder how you could ever have ignored them. You will also be aware of the significance of these changes, and of when you are fertile and infertile.

How effective is the mucus method?

It has been confirmed in laboratory tests that 'the woman's own awareness of her cervical mucus could indicate ovulation even more accurately than [serum] oestrogen measurements'. The effectiveness of the mucus method, correctly applied, for contraception is usually assessed as around 98.5 per cent, but with good teaching and moti-vation rises to 99.8 per cent. However, if you had no experience of using natural methods of contraception before your pregnancy, when your cycles were probably more predictable, you will need to be extra cautious in their application until your cycle has settled down into a regular pattern.

The mucus method is sometimes called the Billings method in honour of the two Australian doctors, Evelyn and John Billings, who pioneered its research and use.

What if your mucus isn't normal?

If your mucus discharge changes in quantity and quality, it is probably your natural cervical mucus, produced in response to hormonal messages. If your mucus is constant, and does not go through changes, has an offensive smell or causes irritation, itching or burning, then you may have an infection and will not be able to rely on the mucus method for contraception. (Of course you should never consider conception while you have an infection.)

If the infection is thrush (candida) or bacterial in origin, it may respond to the following treatment, though do not douche if it is fewer than 10 weeks since you gave birth (or if you are pregnant).

Mix 4 drops of *Tea-tree* oil (a strong antifungal and antiseptic agent), plus 2 tablespoons of white vinegar (to re-acidify) in one litre of warm purified water. Don't use the vinegar if you have any cuts or abrasions. You can douche, bathe (in a sitz-bath, basin or bath) or soak a tampon in the mixture, depending on whether the infection is internal or external. Never leave a tampon in place for longer than eight hours or you could suffer toxic shock syndrome. The amount of solution required will vary according to the method used (you obviously don't need as much in which to dunk your tampon as you do in which to sit). Keep the proportions the same.

Creams and lotions containing *Tea-tree* oil will soothe external itching and irritation. *Tea-tree* pessaries, if available, will help the internal symptoms. Acidophilus yoghurt (live culture) can also work well. It may be taken internally or used locally, and will also help to kill pathogens and re-acidify the vagina. Acidophilus and Bifidus powders or capsules will help to replenish the healthy, yeast-gobbling bacteria that you need when the yeast (thrush) has got out of control.

Garlic is another good immune stimulant. It is strongly antibacterial and antifungal, can be taken internally in large doses and can even be inserted into the vagina. A *Garlic* oil capsule or a clove of garlic, carefully peeled so that it isn't nicked and wrapped in gauze with a tail you can pull then dipped in vegetable oil, can be inserted as a pessary (change it every eight hours), or you can douche with the following herbs: *Golden Seal* (antibacterial), *Uva Ursi* (disinfectant), *Witch Hazel* (astringent to repel pathogens) and *Calendula* (antibacterial and antifungal).

Glycerine makes a good base for a douche if the infection is bacterial (though not for thrush), and you can add a few drops of *Tea-tree* oil for its strong antifungal and antibacterial properties. Use equal parts of all the herbs and glycerine, and always add white vinegar to help re-acidify the vagina.

Intercourse should be avoided, as it spreads the infection back and forth between partners (you should both be treated), or make sure you use condoms. Semen is alkaline, and will encourage infections. If your partner needs treatment, he can use the same herbs and treatments as you. Instead of douching, he can dunk.

If the condition does not respond, you should have a diagnosis carried out by a health practitioner. If you have recurrent candida infections, you will need to investigate the possibility that you are suffering from candida systemically (in the gut).

A great many drugs can also affect mucus production. We have seen how the pill causes the mucus to become infertile, but this is not the only medication which causes problems. Some antibiotics, antihistamines and, ironically, some drugs used to treat infertility can have effects on the production of fertile mucus (more information on this can be found in *Natural Fertility*).

Other conditions which can affect mucus production include:

- dilation and curettage
- thyroid dysfunction
- stress
- cervical problems (erosion, dysplasia, and some of the harsh treatments used to treat these)
- vaginal lubricants, deodorants, douches, sprays or spermicides of a chemical nature, which can cause inflammation of the vaginal lining, or an allergic reaction
- retained tampons
- ovarian disease

As with infection, if your mucus is affected by any of these substances or conditions, you will not be able to use the mucus method for contraception.

Temperature readings and fertility

Temperature readings, although they do not warn of the approach to ovulation like the mucus observations, can still be extremely useful. This is particularly true while you are learning how to tell when you are fertile, and the method is an ideal back-up if there are times of confusion in mucus checking. You can confirm through checking your temperature graph whether or not ovulation has occurred, and if you have entered into the post-ovulatory infertile phase of higher temperatures. If you have previous experience of this method it will help you to recognise a 'lower' and 'higher' range of temperatures, but your readings may be slightly higher overall when breastfeeding than they were before conception.

Mucus observations, and their usefulness in identifying fertile times, can be compromised in a number of situations, as we have seen. Furthermore, even though mucus changes will still be evident, you may be less confident in the first few months, and if any of the following occurs:

- your mucus pattern is different from how it used to be before pregnancy

- it varies from cycle to cycle (due to changing levels of hormones)
- your cycle is irregular
- your level of sexual activity increases

How does temperature reading work?

As ovulation occurs, the increased production of progesterone generates greater heat in the body, and the basal, or body-at-rest, temperature rises. This is what is measured to ascertain whether or not ovulation is over, and when it occurred. It's also why you felt so hot while you were pregnant, when progesterone levels are even higher.

In a classic graph, the temperature jogs along with small changes in the first half, or pre-ovulatory phase, of the menstrual cycle. It drops significantly just before ovulation (this is not always recorded on the graph, as it is a 12-hour drop, and a 24-hour reading), and then rises by up to 0.5°C or 1°F, and stays up until just before, or during, the menstrual period, when it falls again. If ovulation doesn't occur, your temperature won't go up. If menstruation doesn't occur, your temperature won't come down again.

If your body-at-rest temperature has been elevated for more than 20 days, you can consider yourself pregnant. Let's hope that this doesn't

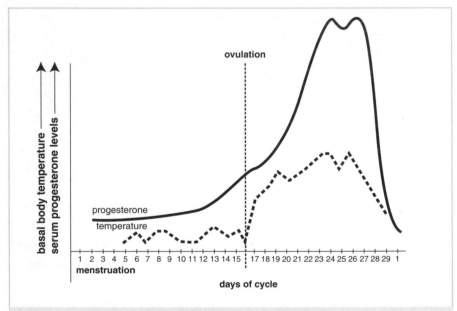

Hormone and basal body temperature levels

happen until about two years after your baby is born, that you have completed your preconception health care, and that this is good news.

At which temperature does ovulation occur?

Ovulation is generally considered to have occurred at the beginning of the temperature rise. This is usually also the lowest reading; your temperature drops by 0.12–0.3°C or 0.25–6°F just before ovulation takes place. However, as we have just noted, this drop may not show on your graph. Therefore, we define the most likely day of ovulation as being at the beginning of the rise, which is not always the lowest temperature *recorded* in the cycle.

Although this is the most likely time for ovulation, it may reasonably commonly occur up to three days prior to the rise. It is also possible for the egg to have been released up to five days before the rise, during the rise, or up to two days after. A late rise may indicate a sluggish progesterone response, which should be treated. Below is a diagram showing the possibilities.

Given good tuition, temperature graphs are easy to interpret after a little experience, and most people can tell from their very first chart when they have finished ovulating, and are therefore infertile.

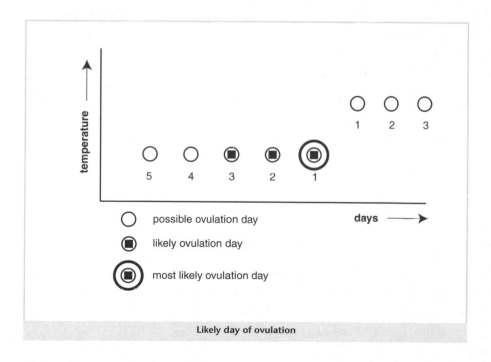

Likely day of ovulation

How to use temperature observations while you are waiting for your cycle to return

It may be unnecessary to take your temperature all the time before your cycle returns, as you may be waiting for your first ovulation for up to a couple of years, so the best plan is to start to take it as soon as you notice any change from the Basic Infertile Pattern of mucus, to see if this results in an ovulation or not. If it does, you can expect a period approximately two weeks later.

How to take your temperature

- The temperature you need to take is your body-at-rest temperature. This means taking it as soon as you wake, before you get out of bed.

- Your temperature should be taken before undertaking any activity. If your baby wakes you and you need to get out of bed, do so gently, get back into bed with him, put him to the breast and take your temperature. If he's in bed with you, less activity will be required, but always note on your graph that activity occurred.

- At least four hours sleep is required to reach the body-at-rest state required. If your baby wakes during the night, and this is a regular pattern, it won't matter. But if your night is more disturbed than usual, mark this on your graph, as your temperature may be raised and you'll need to ignore that day's reading.

- Your temperature should always be taken at the same time of day, as the basal temperature rises through the day. If you wake earlier than usual, adjust the temperature up by 0.05°C (0.1°F) for every half hour before recording it. If later, adjust it down by 0.05°C (0.1°F) for every half hour.

- Other factors which can affect your body-at-rest temperature include ill health, especially fever, and flying across time zones. These occurrences should be noted on your charts.

- We recommend using a mercury thermometer (they are more reliable for small changes than digital), and taking your temperature in the mouth. (We usually find taking your vaginal temperature to be unnecessary.)

How effective is the temperature method?

The temperature method is really very simple to use and can give you some idea of what is going on while you learn to distinguish mucus changes, or if these are unclear. It will also give you information about the timing of ovulation and whether or not this is, in fact, occurring. This information will be invaluable in helping you to know whether your cycles have become ovulatory, and whether your mucus changes precede a real ovulation or just one of those 'now you see me, now you don't' hiccoughs that may occur before your cycle really resumes, as well as helping you to avoid conception. You cannot, however, use the temperature method to warn of the approach of ovulation and, therefore, used alone, it has limited application.

However, the effective rate of the temperature method for contraception correctly applied with abstinence in the pre-ovulatory phase has been assessed as 99 per cent.

If you are using a combination of mucus and temperature observations, which may be further combined with the recording of other cyclical symptoms, the method is called the sympto-thermal method.

There is one other method that you may also be interested to learn about, and use for avoiding conception. This is the observance of a biorhythm, called the lunar cycle, which affects fertility. For reasons that appear below we strongly recommend that in addition to observing your mucus and taking your temperature to confirm ovulation you use protection (or observe abstinence) at your 'lunar peak' times from the time your child is born if you wish to avoid conception.

The lunar cycle

In the 1950s a Czech doctor, Eugen Jonas, identified and assessed a biorhythmic cycle as having an effect upon fertility. Through extensive research and thorough testing, he concluded that a woman is fertile during the same phase of the lunar month that was present when she was born, regardless of whether she is at her mid-cycle ovulation.

This seemingly impossible finding has been extensively tested by both Dr Jonas and many other practitioners and researchers, and some possible answers as to why this may be the case have to do with the moon's relationship with and effect on gravity, ionisation, electro-magnetic fields and light, and the effects these have on a woman's reproductive system.

Several researchers have established that this biorhythm is like a blueprint for the hormonal cycle, and that the more relaxed and generally and reproductively healthy a woman is, the more likely she is to experience her mid-cycle ovulation at the same phase of the moon that was present at her birth. Furthermore, it appears that if this is the case, then her fertility is enhanced, and she is more likely to conceive.

This synchronisation of the hormonal and lunar cycles appears to occur even more readily in women who are aware of their bodies, such as those who are checking their mucus symptoms, or those who are trying to conceive.

It is not surprising that the hormonal cycle has a lunar beat—the word 'menstruation' is derived from classical roots meaning month and moon—and many cultures worldwide have a history of acknowledging the connection between the moon, women and fertility in their religious, mythical and social traditions. An average menstrual cycle is 29.5 days long—the length of a lunar month from one new or full moon to the next.

However, if your menstrual cycle is not regularly this long, it may not synchronise with this lunar blueprint, and the lunar peak may not coincide with ovulation. In these cases, Jonas found that women were often still able to conceive at the lunar peak. In clinical practice, we have also found that conceptions frequently result from intercourse at this time, in situations where the couple is quite confident that no sexual activity occurred at, or near, mid-cycle.

Spontaneous ovulation

How can this be so? Although there is, as yet, no definitive research, the indications are that it may have to do with what is called a spontaneous ovulation. Many studies have confirmed that women can ovulate out of cycle as a response to sexual stimulation. (Ovulation can be assessed in a laboratory by measuring the electrical potential in the body, which increases significantly at ovulation.) It would be interesting to know whether those women were at their lunar peak.

Clinical observations, however, show symptoms normally associated with ovulation (such as changes in cervical mucus and body-at-rest temperature, and ovarian pain) often occur at the lunar peak, even when this does not coincide with the regular, mid-cycle ovulation. Many conceptions have also been recorded by researchers as resulting from intercourse occurring at this time.

How to use the lunar cycle for contraception

Although there are many unanswered questions surrounding this biorhythm and its effect on fertility, it is difficult to ignore the extensive findings and therefore the need to take them into account for contraceptive purposes. The angle between the sun and the moon present at the time of the woman's birth needs to be calculated, and then the dates of the return of this angle each lunar month must be predicted. These times can then be used as a guide for avoiding conception, given certain guidelines and safety margins for egg and sperm life. Briefly, this involves abstaining from using barrier methods of contraception for 3½ days before the recurrence of the natal sun/moon angle (to allow for sperm lifespan) and 12 hours afterwards (to allow for the lifespan of the egg).

If you wish to use this cycle to increase your chances of avoiding conception, it is obviously preferable and easier if the biorhythmic and hormonal cycles synchronise, creating one fertile time per month. This can be achieved, in many cases, by fulfilling the conditions known to predispose women to ovulating at this lunar peak. These include becoming reproductively and generally healthy, less stressed, avoiding activities (such as air travel across time zones) known to disrupt cycles, and becoming aware of the body changes associated with the hormonal cycle. It is also helpful to be aware of the individual lunar cycle, as this will influence the timing of your hormonal cycle in much the same way as women who live together ovulate and menstruate at the same time as each other. Visualisation and affirmation techniques can also be used to great effect.

How to use the lunar cycle while you are waiting for your cycle to return

Until your cycle has resumed a regular pattern, it's obviously not possible for your hormonal and lunar cycles to synchronise. This means that you will need to observe abstinence or protection for the whole 4 days at all your lunar peak times in order to avoid the possibility of a spontaneous ovulation, to which some women seem to be particularly prone. Just to emphasise why we think that's important, we should tell you that all the conceptions that we've known about during all our years of practice that occurred within a few weeks of birth seemed to result from unprotected intercourse taking place at a lunar peak time. You must consider your lunar peak days fertile from two weeks after childbirth, because a spontaneous ovulation will not be preceded by mucus changes, and there will be no warning.

HOW TO LEARN NATURAL CONTRACEPTION

The methods of natural contraception we've outlined are widely taught. They may be described as 'Natural Family Planning', 'Natural Birth Control' or 'Natural Fertility Awareness'. We prefer the term 'Natural Fertility Management', implying the use of the same methods for both avoiding and achieving conception, and for identifying reproductive and menstrual problems which can then be remedied using natural medicine.

Natural Fertility Management is a system developed by Francesca that includes the use of mucus and temperature methods, rhythm calculations (where appropriate) and lunar cycle observance. It is widely taught by health professionals trained by Francesca in its use. You can learn to use these methods by contacting us for the name of one of our counsellors, or for a mail-order kit. This kit includes tapes, notes, charts, computer-calculated lunar biorhythms and Francesca's book *Natural Fertility*, which comprehensively explains the use of the methods (see Recommended Reading and Contacts and Resources).

There are several other aids that can be bought that help you detect your fertile period. Some of these test body-at-rest temperature, and some the surge in luteinising hormone (LH) that precedes ovulation.

Clear Plan, The Right Day, and First Response are all kits available through pharmacies which measure the LH surge by testing the urine. Most kits come with sufficient assessment indications to last one or two cycles. They are rather expensive to use on a regular basis, but can be useful if you are confused about your mucus or temperature observations. Baby-comp and Lady-comp are computer-assisted thermometers which build up a record of your temperature observations and claim to be able to predict the fertile time in advance. They will only work for regular cycles, and so may not be useful during breastfeeding.

Another quite useful device is a microscope that lets you see if your mucus is 'ferning', which is the pattern to which most fertile mucus crystallises as it dries on a slide. Since saliva is also affected by hormones, it will show the same effect. You can buy microscopes that are especially designed for the purpose, and, although not cheap, they are reuseable so the cost may be defrayed over several cycles. They can provide a helpful adjunct to manual testing and your awareness of the sensation of the mucus. However, in our opinion, they do not replace the look-and-feel approach.

STAYING CONFIDENT UNTIL YOU'RE READY FOR YOUR NEXT CONCEPTION

You'll find that natural contraception methods serve you well while you're breastfeeding, as long as you're diligent. Mucus observations will always warn you of an approaching ovulation (and if by any chance there's not any mucus, then the sperm can't survive and you are not fertile even if you ovulate). The temperature method will confirm if you have ovulated or not, and therefore if you should expect a period two weeks later. Your lunar peak times should always be observed, and you may notice symptoms of ovarian activity at these times. However, the use of these methods is not restricted to the time that you're breast-feeding. They are methods that you can continue to use for fertility management throughout your fertile life, either for contraception, or to help plan your next 'conscious' conception.

10

Common problems for breastfeeding mothers

ILLNESS WHILE YOU'RE BREASTFEEDING

In most cases, even if you are quite ill, you can continue breastfeeding. In fact, it's important that you do so, as your baby's best protection comes through your milk. There are some diseases that will require that you stop, and you'll find those in Appendix 3. You should always seek medical advice, but it's quite possible to go on feeding even though, for example, you may have a bad case of the 'flu and a raging temperature. The protection your baby receives from your milk is much more important than any concerns you have of contagion—and in most cases infections are passed in the early stages, before you're even aware of being ill.

However, it's important to get help. Don't try to soldier on—if you do you could risk your milk supply. If you're not trying to attend to family and home as well as your breastfeeding baby, you've got a better chance of a quick recovery. If you need prescription drugs, your doctor needs to know that you are breastfeeding. It's also important to make it clear that you are committed to a continuing breastfeeding relationship, and to be sure that your doctor prescribes the drug that is least likely to be transmitted to your baby through the milk. This will depend on the dosage used, the molecular weight of the drug, whether or not it is fat-soluble, how much of the drug is bound to plasma, how quickly it breaks down and how efficiently your body detoxifies and eliminates it. All of these factors will vary considerably, but when a careful, thoughtful choice is made, your baby need be only minimally affected (if at all).

If you, or your doctor, are in any doubt about the safety of a particular medication, research it well, and a lactation consultant will also be able to advise you. Appendix 1 contains information about some classes of prescription and over-the-counter drugs which should be avoided.

Although most drugs pass into your milk, the amount is small, and in many cases will be acceptable. If you need to take medication for a chronic condition the amount of drug transmitted to your baby in utero will have exceeded the amount he receives through your breast milk. If you need to take medication for an acute condition you can reduce the amount that transfers to your milk by taking it immediately after you have fed your baby; there will be a reduced concentration in the milk by the next time you feed. For this reason, it's best to avoid long-acting or slow-release medications, since they are delivered to the body over a long period of time. Ask your doctor to prescribe the fast-acting form.

If you need to have antibiotic treatment, you will need to take acidophilus and bifidus lactobacilli, available in supplement form (powders or capsules) from your health food shop, to replace your gut flora—these lactobacilli will also be present, in lesser concentrations, in cultured, natural yoghurt. You may also need to feed some yoghurt to your baby if he develops digestive problems. No matter what the medication, monitor your baby at all times for adverse reactions and monitor your milk supply too. Don't be afraid to ask your doctor to review your medication schedule if you are concerned about your baby or your supply. There's always more than one drug that can be used to treat any condition and it might simply mean a bit of trial and error until you get the right drug (or combination) that suits both of you.

If you visit a naturopath or herbalist, you are more likely to receive treatment that won't affect your baby, but they also need to be told that you are breastfeeding. There's a list of contraindicated (and safe) herbs in Appendix 2. If you follow any of our recommended treatments, you can be confident that the herbs and other natural remedies we recommend are safe to use. Appendix 5 will give you instructions on how to apply the remedies we suggest.

RELACTATION

If your illness is such that you can't breastfeed, or you are unavoidably separated from your baby for a time, don't despair, it doesn't mean that your milk supply and your chances of breastfeeding are gone forever. You can relactate when you and your baby are reunited or when you've recovered (if you had to stop because of illness). Relactation may take up to 10 days and will be most successful when you take your baby into your bed and let him feed almost constantly. Make sure that you've got help in the house so that you can focus on building up your milk supply without the stress of attending to the rest of the family.

If you are told you need to stop feeding for any reason, always try to get a second opinion (from a lactation consultant, for example) and try to limit the time to as few days as possible. You may be able to express your milk and have it fed to your baby (and though it's not normally a problem, you'd need to be sure that infection couldn't be passed on this way). See the section on expressing milk in Chapter 4. If you can't use expressed milk, then see Chapter 8 for alternatives—using goat's milk with added acidophilus and bifidus lactobacilli is probably the best— and it's preferable, if you are planning to return to the breast, to use a cup or spoon, not a bottle.

FEEDING MORE THAN ONE BABY

If you're the mother of twins or other multiples, or if you're facing the prospect of nursing your baby as well as your toddler, you need to be especially aware of all the ways of ensuring that your milk supply is up to the task (see Chapter 4). You'll need to pay extra special attention to your diet and your supplementation program (see Chapter 5) as well as all the other factors that contribute to breastfeeding success (see Chapters 3, 6 and 7). A good support network is vital, especially in the early days, particularly if your nursing babies are multiples rather than siblings. However, the law of supply and demand seems to work just as well for two (or even three) babies as it does for one, which is just as well as twins can often be quite small at birth and have an even greater need for the best nourishment on offer.

If you are nursing twins, triplets (or even more babies), and if it's the first time you've breastfed, it's probably easier to feed one baby at a time. This way you can ensure a correct latch and each baby will get a full feed of foremilk and hindmilk. If your babies are anxious for the breast at the same time, a support person can help while you stay relaxed to feed one. As you and the babies get the hang of it, you can sit in a chair with cushions supporting your arms and with two babies in your lap nursing simultaneously. Some mothers find it easier to tuck their babies under their arms.

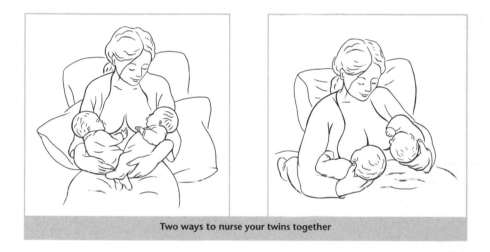

Two ways to nurse your twins together

An older child will often wean himself if you're nursing through a pregnancy, especially when your milk changes to colostrum. However if he doesn't (and it's often easier if he continues to nurse, especially if the births are closely spaced) you'll still need to give your new baby the chance to latch on properly and get his feeding routine established. Even if you're an old hand at the game, always make sure that your new baby's needs are met before your toddler's. However, tandem nursing can be a wonderful way to defuse any sibling rivalry and gives you some time when you can really focus on your new baby while still responding to the needs of your older child.

TOO MUCH MILK

If you worry that your baby isn't getting enough milk, you might wonder how an over-abundant supply could ever be considered a problem. But some women do feel like jersey cows. Their clothes, bedding, baby and partner are constantly saturated and their babies gasp and choke as they try to cope with veritable fountains of milk. Francesca often wondered whether she should set herself up as a public fountain—but thought that might be taking the earth-mother thing too far!

If over-supply is a problem for you, you should always feed your baby from the least full breast to avoid him being overwhelmed by the flow. If you're well co-ordinated, ambidextrous and have the energy and inclination, take the opportunity to collect the milk that flows from the fuller breast while you nurse your baby at the other. To do this, you should use a sterile nipple shield and a sterile bottle. Try to avoid stimulating the breast when collecting the milk, as this will increase supply. You can add to the refrigerated supply in the bottle at any time in 24 hours, after which you'll have to transfer the bottle to the freezer in the fridge (store for 2 weeks) or to a deep-freeze where it can be stored for up to 3 months. Then, without any effort, you have a supply of breast milk for emergencies, or for when you can't be there for your baby. If you've got a really copious supply you might consider donating some to a hospital milk bank (although we wish you luck in finding one).

If you need to relieve a very full breast between feeds, apply a hot cloth or compress and allow the milk to flow until the discomfort is relieved. Don't express more milk than is absolutely necessary to give you relief; you'll only stimulate the production of more. One way of slowing down the flow is to hold and press the areola between your fingers while you're feeding. This may take a little practice, but may work better than lying on your back, which is often suggested. Sucking against gravity can be a problem for your baby unless the flow of milk is particularly strong.

An old folk remedy for reducing flow is to apply fresh *Jasmine* flowers to the breast. The fresh flowers can be held on to the breast with adhesive tape. Take great care, however, not to reduce your supply too much and don't use the essential oil, which is stronger in its action. *Jasmine* affects prolactin levels which is why we told you in Chapter 4 to avoid it, unless you're trying to wean. As with *Jasmine*, we also warned you to avoid *Sage*. A small amount of *Sage* tea, however, may be just the trick to reduce excessive flow. Just be careful not to overdo it. You may also find it helpful to have your baby in a semi-upright position, with his head tilted well back. In this position, he'll be more able to cope with the fast flow.

Fortunately for both you and your baby, this over-abundant supply usually settles down to a more manageable level within four weeks of the birth. However this doesn't mean that your supply is diminishing. You can also be comforted by the fact that when your milk flows freely like this, the chances of suffering from blocked ducts or mastitis are remote.

MASTITIS, BLOCKED DUCTS AND ENGORGEMENT

If you're unfortunate enough to suffer from mastitis, you might well wish that you'd had to deal with an over-supply of milk instead. Mastitis is an inflammation of the breast tissue. It's often diagnosed as an infection, but that's not necessarily the case. It can be caused by such apparently innocent situations as an over-tight bra or car seatbelt, or pressure from a handbag strap or from your arm while you sleep. The most common cause, however, is incomplete drainage of the ducts, which usually occurs because your baby isn't positioned correctly. If one of the small milk-carrying tubules becomes kinked, twisted or compressed (it's a little like putting a kink in a hose), protein molecules will diffuse into the surrounding tissue, causing inflammation and mastitis.

The first symptom is a sore red patch which grows and intensifies until your breast is exquisitely painful, hot to touch and as hard as a lump of concrete. As if that's not enough, you'll have a temperature, a headache and a bout of 'flu-like symptoms that will send you off to bed.

And that's just where you need to stay. Take your baby with you and feed him constantly and exclusively from the affected breast (too little feeding or incomplete drainage may well have caused the problem in the first place). If there is a particularly sore spot resulting from a blocked duct, get him to feed with his chin pointing towards it and always make sure he is correctly positioned and attached. If your breasts are both engorged, or there is no infection or inflammation, you can let him feed from both breasts, but make sure each breast is completely drained before offering the other.

You can also use hot compresses, a hot-water bottle or a hot shower with the water jet directed on the affected area. Massage towards your nipple with almond or apricot kernel oil. (In the case of venous engorgement that can occur in the first few days after birth, use cold compresses and cold showers.) While these natural remedies will be painful at the start, they're preferable to the use of antibiotics that may not only be unnecessary, but will play havoc with the intestinal flora in both you and your baby. If you need to take antibiotics, follow our advice earlier in this chapter. If you need painkillers, paracetamol is preferable to aspirin, which is better avoided during lactation.

Increasing the circulation of blood to the affected area can also help: activities such as a game of tennis, scrubbing or polishing the floor and wringing out nappies by hand are all guaranteed (and indeed suggested) to improve blood flow. Since only a complete sadist would suggest that you attempt any of these while you're suffering from mastitis, below are a few other natural remedies for sore, engorged or infected breasts that you might prefer to try. (In the case of venous engorgement during the first few days after birth, blood flow needs to be reduced, so stay still and relaxed. You're not likely to want to play tennis then anyway!)

- Try to leave your bra off as often as possible.

- Drink lots of fluids: at least a glass of purified water every hour (but not iced, even if you feel hot).

- Apply a poultice, compress or ointment of *Poke Root*, *Comfrey*, *Parsley*, *Witch Hazel*, *Chamomile*, *Burdock*, *Ginger*, *Slippery Elm*, *Marshmallow Root* or the essential oils *Geranium*, *Rose*, *Chamomile* and *Lavender*. A compress can be made by soaking a face flannel in an infusion of the herb (see Appendix 5), or in water sprinkled with a few drops of the oils. Make sure you wash your breast very thoroughly before your baby next feeds.

- *Hypericum* oil (not an essential oil) can be made by covering the fresh leaves and flowers of *St John's Wort* with vegetable oil (olive oil is good) and exposing it to the sun for six weeks. Make sure the oil completely covers the plant to stop it growing mould. *St John's Wort* provides relief for pain as well as inflammation. Apply the oil directly to the breast, or in a compress. *Hypericum* oil may be available in your health food shop. Wash it off thoroughly before the next feed.

※ Put bruised or steamed *Cabbage* or *Comfrey* leaves in your bra, or a poultice of raw mashed potato (very tasty . . . and sexy to boot!). You can bruise the cabbage leaves with a rolling pin. Use them cold from the fridge for engorgement in the first few feeding days, but warm them for mastitis or blocked ducts. Discard after 20 minutes or, if using them cold, when they warm up.

※ For a cold compress, put some ice cubes in a plastic bag and wrap it all up in a cloth nappy or towel.

※ Massage the reflex zones for the breasts and the axillary lymphatics. (see pp. 48 & 65)

※ Massage the breast towards the nipple (from behind any particularly sore spots) while your baby feeds. This encourages the milk to flow down any blocked ducts.

※ Rotate your arms backwards (as if swimming on your back) to help drain excess fluid from your breasts.

※ If your breasts are swollen and lumpy with pain radiating all over your body, take the homoeopathic version of *Poke Root* internally. This remedy is called *Phytolacca*. *Poke Root* is too toxic to take in herbal form while you're breastfeeding. (See Appendix 5 for general information on homoeopathy.)

※ Other helpful homoeopathic remedies are *Belladonna* (for too much milk with breasts that are hot, swollen, rock hard and tender to touch), *Bryonia* (if your breasts are hot and painful) and *Sulphur* (if there is infection or if your nipples smart and burn after feeding).

※ Herbs to take internally for infection include *Echinacea*, *St John's Wort* (this is better supervised by a herbalist when breastfeeding) and *Red Clover* (for a short time only as it contains phyto-oestrogens). *Garlic* is also a good immune stimulant.

✗ In the case of fever, *Lime Flowers* or *Elder Flowers* (or both) should be taken as a hot tea (see Appendix 5). Stay warm under the covers and sweat it out.

✗ You may find it helpful to increase your intake of vitamins A and E temporarily. Vitamin A can be taken in doses up to 30 000 IU daily (for no more than 1–2 weeks) and vitamin E in doses up to 1000 IU daily.

✗ Up to 4 grams of vitamin C daily, in divided doses every 2–3 hours, can be important in fighting infection. Though this may give your baby diarrhoea (as may the larger doses of *Garlic)*, this may be less of a problem than your infection. However, you must keep feeding him to avoid dehydration.

If these treatments help, you may be able to avoid using medication. If, however, the condition seems to be worsening at each feed, consult a doctor straight away. To avoid a recurrence of the condition, you should avoid the situations that lead to tubules becoming blocked or compressed. A bra that fits poorly or is too tight, sleeping on an overly full breast and going too long between feeds can all lead to the development of blocked ducts or mastitis.

CRACKED, SORE OR RETRACTED NIPPLES

Nipples that are tender, sore, painful, bruised, stinging or aching aren't an incentive to breastfeed, and may cause (as well as be caused by) poor breastfeeding habits or technique. They may be sore on the first few days of nursing (especially if you're fair-skinned), though good preparation before the birth can be very helpful. See Chapter 3 for more on preparation, and remember that adequate zinc status promotes strong nipple tissue (see Chapter 5 for ways to ensure you're getting enough zinc).

By far the best way to avoid traumatised nipples is to make sure your baby is positioned and latched on correctly (see Chapter 3). Remember, it's best if you're both naked. Your baby should face you with his chest against yours. His head should rest on your arm and his chin should nestle at the base of your breast ('Chest to chest, chin to breast'). Point his nose towards your nipple and make sure his mouth is wide open so that he can get a good latch on the areola as well as the nipple. The nipple should be free inside his mouth (if you suck your thumb you'll see what we mean), and he should not be pulling on the nipple, or the breast, so make sure his head is at a good height.

If he is not attached properly, he won't get a good flow of milk and, in his frustration, will suck harder and harder, making the problem worse. If you think he's not latched on properly, don't pull him off your breast (ouch!), but detach him gently by releasing the suction with your finger (see Chapter 3 again). Then start again. Sore nipples are *not* caused by letting your baby suck for too long, as was once thought. In fact, as we've already discussed, the hindmilk is of great benefit to your baby. So continue to feed fully and often to avoid your baby getting too hungry between feeds and consequently attaching aggressively.

It's also important, as preventative care, to look after your breasts and nipples. Some of the measures we mentioned in Chapter 3 as preparation also apply here. Keep your nipples clean and dry, avoid soap and use non-abrasive natural fibre bras. Expose your breasts and nipples to fresh air and sunlight whenever possible. (Although we're staunch advocates of breastfeeding in public, we'd advise you to restrict this airing and sunbathing to your home or the beach!) If going without a bra is too uncomfortable, leave the flaps in your maternity bra open after feeding. Change wet bras and shirts as soon as you can, and take care with breast pads that have plastic backing (this holds moisture against the nipple). A moist condition can encourage yeast infection (candida), which can be a major problem (more on this shortly).

However, if your nipples are already sore or cracked, you'll need some remedies and treatment for the acute phase of the condition while you're attending to the preventative measures above.

- If you're feeling apprehensive about feeding, you may tense up. This will inhibit your let-down reflex, your baby won't receive a good flow and then he will suck harder. Use any of the techniques we suggested in Chapter 4 to help you relax before and during nursing.

- Encourage the let-down reflex before you start feeding to reduce the time your baby spends at the breast sucking on an empty nipple. Hand-expressing, warm water or towels, warm drinks and even just thinking about a (pleasurable) feeding experience will help. Wait for the tingle that accompanies let-down, then put him to your breast.

❧ Feed from the less sore side first, when your baby is more energetic. If the soreness is really severe, you may need to only feed from one side for a whole day, while you treat the other nipple. In extreme cases, you may even need to express your milk and give it to your baby with a spoon, cup or dropper until your nipples have recovered.

❧ To encourage air flow around your nipples and keep the fabric of your bra or shirt from rubbing on them, you can buy two tea-strainers, cut off the handles and cup the domed mesh over your nipples, inside your bra cup.

❧ An ice block applied to the nipple before feeding can partially numb it and reduce the level of pain you experience.

❧ Smearing the fatty hindmilk onto your nipple at the end of a feed protects and encourages healing and discourages infection, as it contains antibodies.

❧ The cabbage leaf we mentioned for mastitis can also be used for sore nipples. Not only does it help healing, but it's softer against your nipple than most bras.

❧ Herbs which can soften and soothe sensitive nipples include *Calendula, Comfrey, Chickweed, St John's Wort, Aloe Vera, Yarrow* and *Squaw Vine*. They can be applied as an ointment, cream or poultice. *St John's Wort* can also be applied as *Hypericum* oil (see 'Mastitis') and *Aloe Vera* as a gel. Make sure to wash them off the whole breast carefully before the next feed.

❧ *Lavender* and *Rose* essential oils can soothe sore nipples. Use a very dilute mixture of one drop in a teaspoon of nut or olive oil and massage directly into your nipples after each feed. Remember to wash the whole areola and nipple thoroughly before the next feed.

❧ Even plain olive or almond oil can help. Some women find that pure lanolin (not toilet lanolin which is more commonly available) is preferable, with or without herbs or essential oils added, though it can (rarely) cause an allergic reaction. Vitamin E cream and even honey (which has antimicrobial properties) can also be effective (though should be washed off before the next feed). We've also known women to get results from applying the Bach flower remedy *Rescue Remedy* to the affected nipple.

- *Garlic, Propolis, Echinacea, Golden Seal, Myrrh* and vitamin C are helpful to take internally and apply topically if there's an infection. This is especially likely if the nipples are cracked, providing an entry point for bacteria. If your baby gets diarrhoea, you may need to reduce the dose of vitamin C.

- Homoeopathic remedies for sore or cracked nipples include *Chamomilla* (for inflamed and very tender nipples), *Lycopodium* (for cracked nipples that bleed during feeds), *Staphysagria* (for extreme nipple pain when feeding), *Causticum, Graphites* and *Silica*. It's best to consult with a professional homoeopath to get the correct remedy.

- As well as the reflexology areas for the breast (direct and indirect), you can pay special attention to the nipple point.

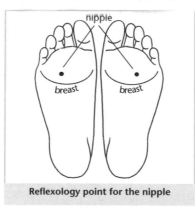

Reflexology point for the nipple

- If your nipples are cracked, you may need to stop feeding from that breast until the cracks have healed. You shouldn't use ointments or creams during this time, but you can apply the fluid extract or tincture of the appropriate helpful herbs directly. Use the ointments after the cracks have dried up.

- In severe cases, or if your nipple is retracted (drawn back into your breast), you may find it helpful to use a nipple shield. The use of these is controversial, as they can interfere with the stimulation you need to produce milk, but the newer versions, made from silica, are thinner and less problematic. The smaller shields designed for newborns may also be more successful. They should only be used short-term so milk production can continue successfully, and can be obtained from pharmacies. Ask your lactation counsellor for help in using these successfully.

- If your nipple is retracted, inverted or flat, your baby will find it more difficult to latch on and the frustration cycle begins. If he gets too angry, don't persist. Detach him, soothe him and start again. Massage your nipple between finger and thumb to draw it out, and press the areola into a flatter shape.

- For really severe cases, especially if there is infection, seek medical help. You may need to use an antibiotic cream if the measures we suggest here aren't adequate. If so, make sure you clean it off well before feeds, as it will affect your baby's gut flora if he ingests it.

FOOD ALLERGIES

Allergy means compromised nutritional status

If you have an allergic profile your nutritional status will be compromised. A food allergy can impair absorption of essential minerals and vitamins, and other nutrients are used up as your body tries to restore itself to balance and good health. Obviously this can affect your health and, consequently, that of your baby. One of the reasons we recommend nutritional supplements is to make up for the deficits which might be due to an allergic condition.

If you are allergic or intolerant to the common allergens listed below (or to other foods), then your baby may also react to the same foods. While your child shares the nourishment that your body provides, he also shares your allergic responses. The more frequent or severe your responses are, the more likely it is that he will be vulnerable to these same responses. Colic is a very common reaction, but other gastro-intestinal problems, skin conditions and respiratory problems, including ear, nose and throat infections, may also be due to an allergic response. Before you can solve the problem of your baby's allergic response, you need to deal with your own allergies.

How to identify allergens

Some common food allergens include cow's milk dairy products, beef, wheat (and rye, oats and corn), eggs (and chicken meat), citrus fruits, pork, peanuts, yeast, cane and beet sugar, and food additives such as colourings and preservatives. If you suspect that food allergies or sensi-tivities are a problem for you, and therefore for your baby, there are several very simple and safe tests described below which you can administer yourself to identify the culprits. However, provocation testing, which involves introducing a sample of the suspected substance and observing the reaction, and elimination diets are best avoided while you're breastfeeding.

Which food do you crave?

First of all you could ask yourself which food you crave. If you can identify a food which you believe you simply could not live without, then that food is frequently the offender.

Keeping a food diary

An extremely simple way to identify allergens is to start keeping a record of the foods you've eaten in the 6-, 12- and 24-hour periods that have preceded adverse symptoms that you might experience or those, such as constant crying, that your baby might exhibit. You might also note any unusual environmental circumstances.

The pulse test

The pulse test is another way to identify problem foods. You simply take your resting pulse then eat a normal portion of the suspect food. After eating, you take your pulse again at 10-minute intervals for an hour, and if it is elevated or lowered by more than 10 beats per minute, the food is likely to be one that is affecting you adversely. Remember not to confuse an increased pulse rate with increased physical activity; make sure you stay relatively quiet while you're applying this test.

Kinesiology (muscle testing)

Another way to easily detect sensitivity or allergy, or even to determine if a food (or condition) is helpful or not, is through kinesiology, or muscle testing. This is best carried out by a trained practitioner, although you can learn to use a simple form quite effectively at home. It can also be used to suggest which treatment would be most effective or which organ or system needs attention. You need to stand erect with one arm extended, level with the shoulder. The practitioner or tester places one hand on your extended arm at the wrist and the other on your opposite shoulder. If you then imagine a strengthening situation (such as eating a bowl of green salad) followed by a weakening situation (such as eating a bowl of white sugar) and the tester presses down firmly on your extended wrist after each visualisation, there should be a detectable difference in resistance—this should show a stronger response (greater resistance) for green salad than for white sugar, as you can safely assume that green salad is beneficial, and white sugar is not.

These two baseline responses can then be used as a benchmark while you imagine (or affirm out loud) that you are eating or experiencing a certain food or situation. Even better, you might hold up the food with your free hand to your thymus area (at the base of your neck above your breast bone), or place a small amount under your tongue. This method of testing is remarkably accurate and generally as reliable as any other method of allergy testing, though much simpler and less expensive!

Dowsing

If your practitioner has experience in using a pendulum (dowsing), he or she may be able to obtain quite accurate clues as to which foods or conditions are affecting you. This can be done by swinging the pendulum over the food (or even over the written name of the food) while maintaining contact with you.

Both muscle testing and dowsing can also be used to ask questions such as, 'How often can I eat this food? Once a week? Every other day?' and, 'How long do I need to abstain from this food? A week? A month?' and so on. This sort of testing can also be used to answer questions of dosage, duration and appropriateness of treatment.

How to deal with allergens

Once you're certain that you or your baby are reacting adversely to something you eat, inhale, touch or are otherwise exposed to, there are several things that we recommend you do.

Avoidance

First of all you should avoid any foods which you know are a definite problem for you. It's often more difficult to avoid airborne allergens such as pollen or dust, but it's important that you do the very best you can. The total avoidance of many foods is extremely difficult, but don't panic! Recent research shows that very occasional exposure to or ingestion of an allergen is even better, in terms of the outcome for your child and his allergic status, than complete abstention, as long as the exposure is limited in amount and frequency.

Maintain a healthy diet and lifestyle

Maintain a healthy diet and avoid pollutants whenever possible. Also use our recommended doses of nutritional supplements throughout the full period of breastfeeding.

Additionally, there are some useful herbs, including *Hemidesmus* and the mushrooms *Reishii* and *Shiitake*, which act as immune system modulators (help to prevent an over-reaction of the immune system), and others (for example, *Albizzia* and *Baical Scullcap*), which reduce allergic response.

Don't eat cow's milk products if you're allergic to them

We certainly don't recommend that you continue to eat an offending food, even if it's generally considered essential for good health. We mention this because many breastfeeding women have a morbid fear of going without cow's milk—they imagine a child with brittle bones and teeth falling from his head. Since milk is by far the most common allergenic food (hardly surprising when it contains hundreds of very reactive phenolic compounds), many of you will be allergic or sensitive to cow's milk and products made from it. Both you and your baby will be better off without these products, since constant consumption can lead to nutritional deficits and a very compromised maternal immune system (and probably a child with a similar allergy).

Now that we've hit you with an iconoclastic statement about avoiding dairy foods our reputations will be mud in orthodox circles, but there are a few relevant facts that might help to reassure you about our recommendation. Minerals such as zinc and magnesium and nutrients such as vitamin A are as equally important as calcium in bone and teeth formation. Magnesium, in fact, is the only mineral which has been demonstrated to increase bone density. Furthermore, calcium is very poorly absorbed from cow's milk, and if you're allergic to cow's milk, that absorption is even further impaired.

We'd also like to remind you that a significant proportion of the world's population cannot tolerate dairy foods, yet manage to obtain all the calcium they need from other sources. Remember, too, that weight-bearing exercise keeps calcium in your bones (see Chapter 7).

Non-cow's milk sources of calcium

There are numerous foods that are good sources of calcium if you cannot tolerate cow's milk. Milk, yoghurt and cheese from goats or sheep, seaweed, collard leaves, beet, dandelion and turnip greens, parsley, watercress, broccoli, spinach, sesame seeds (hulled), tahini paste, almonds, brazil nuts, tofu, ripe olives, cooked soya beans and salmon and sardines with the bones are all good sources of calcium. Of course if there's still some doubt in your mind a supplement containing calcium is your insurance policy. Remember that such a supplement should not be taken alone since it will inhibit the absorption of zinc and iron, but should only be taken as part of our recommended supplementation program (see Chapter 5).

You don't need to avoid problem allergens forever

Once the offending substances have been recognised, it shouldn't be necessary for you to live on a totally restricted diet or in a sterile atmosphere. There is much that can be done using natural medicine to strengthen your immune, digestive and other systems. It should be possible, with an improved diet and lifestyle, and generally strengthened systems, to re-introduce offending dietary substances on a rotating basis. This is preferable to total exclusion.

By dealing effectively with allergens you will improve your general health because the total stress on your immune and other organ systems will be reduced. You'll also give your baby a better chance of nutritional adequacy, a better chance of an immune system which isn't compromised and consequently a better chance of being free from similar allergies and sensitivities to those you have suffered.

CANDIDA

Candida, or thrush, can be a major problem for a breastfeeding mum, as it can infect the breast and cause hot, deep, searing pain deep in the breast during feeding. This pain, and the sore nipples that accompany it, can make you quite disinclined to continue to feed. Your baby may also refuse the breast, even though he appears hungry.

Candida can infect not only the breast, but may also be a problem in the vagina or any other moist, dark environment, such as your baby's mouth. If it occurs repeatedly, it's possible, even likely, that it has become systemic and invaded the gut. Systemic candidiasis is a growing problem, largely resulting from overprescription of antibiotics, the oral contraceptive pill and some other commonly prescribed drugs such as corticosteroids, which disturb intestinal flora, allowing harmful micro-organisms to proliferate. Poor dietary habits such as eating too much sugary food and refined carbohydrates can also cause, or contribute to, the problem.

The most common strain is *Candida albicans* (from alba, meaning white, and reflecting the white curdy discharge common to infected areas). This is normally a benign yeast organism present in the gut (and in all mucous membranes) but held in check by 'good' bacteria. There are also several other strains, with some of the more recently discovered ones proving resistant to antifungal agents and accounting for up to half of the cases of candida currently seen. The systemic condition is frequently undiagnosed, but can be the cause of a great deal of illness, particularly among women.

Vaginal thrush is often experienced during pregnancy, when the high level of circulating hormones creates a favourable environment for its growth. This will be much more likely to occur if you were prone to candida before you conceived, so the best time to treat it is as part of your preconception health care. If vaginal thrush is present during delivery it can infect your baby, who can then infect your breast. And on it goes. A major cause of thrush during breastfeeding can be anti-biotics prescribed for mastitis, so use the natural remedies we advised earlier if you have sore breasts, and see if you can deal with this problem without the use of drugs if possible. Women prescribed the mini-pill while breastfeeding may also have a greater tendency to develop candida, so read Chapter 9 and avoid this drug also. If your baby is prescribed antibiotics for any reason, the chain reaction may start with him.

Is it candida?

There may be a number of reasons for your breasts to be sore (see our earlier suggestions). If they appear red with tiny white spots and flaky skin, if the pain radiates from the nipple, and the nipples are also inflamed, or if they itch, then candida is a probable diagnosis. This is even more likely to be the cause if you have previously had problems with candida (systemic or vaginally), or if your baby has oral thrush. If he's also experiencing diarrhoea or abdominal gas (common side effects), refusing to feed even though he appears hungry, and is fussy and irritable, your suspicions would be further confirmed.

The consistency of oral thrush is quite different to the coating of milk left behind after a feed—it's clottier, coats the tongue and inner cheeks and is not easy to scrape off. Your baby may also have a red flaky rash on his bottom, the crease of his neck and his thighs, and in his armpits. If you have a daughter, she may have white curds in the labial folds. Your red flaky rash may be worse under your breasts where they lie against your chest. You may also be experiencing vaginal thrush, with a discharge which smells yeasty, and intense itching or soreness. Of course, you could be suffering from a different genital infection, and although the yeasty smell would in that case be replaced by one which is more 'fishy', you may need a professional diagnosis to be sure. Vaginal candida is worsened, or triggered, if you wear synthetic underwear or tight trousers, use vaginal deodorants, soaps or detergents, or wipe 'back to front' after a bowel motion. Hot weather will make all forms of thrush worse.

If infections in you or your baby are recurrent or severe, you need to consider whether the condition may be systemic, and infecting your gut (or your baby's).

Diagnosing systemic candida

Intestinal (systemic) candida is more difficult to diagnose, though a naturopath may have some suggestions as there are various techniques and procedures which can help to identify the condition. You may be more likely to suffer from systemic candida if you have used antibiotics recently or frequently, taken the oral contraceptive pill or had a poor diet high in sugar and refined carbohydrates, as these will all act to disturb the delicate balance of 'healthy' bacteria and yeasts in your gut. Symptoms of systemic candida include:

- fatigue
- colic or abdominal pain
- flatulence
- food cravings
- eczema or tinea
- alcohol or sugar cravings or intolerance
- dry flaky skin
- digestive disturbances
- rashes
- depression or anxiety
- difficulty concentrating
- mood swings
- muscle weakness
- poor memory
- nasal congestion
- blurry vision
- headaches
- chronic respiratory infections
- aches and pains
- allergies (especially to yeast and mould)
- cystitis
- itchiness (especially anal)

Treating candida

It's important to diagnose and treat candida as quickly as possible, so you can continue breastfeeding. If it gets too painful and your baby is also rejecting the breast, it can get very difficult. So get professional help if our suggestions don't bring fast relief, as it's important to keep feeding. There are a few things you can do which should ease the condition considerably.

⚘ If your breasts are affected, keep them clean and dry. Because candida thrives in moist, dark environments, don't wear breast pads or nipple shields, take your bra off as much as possible, and leave your breasts open to the air. If your bra or shirt gets wet, change it.

⚘ If your baby has a rash, keep him dry too (especially his bottom). Dust on some *Slippery Elm* powder, especially in the creases, and this will soothe his skin. This is an excellent substitute for talcum powder which can clog his pores. You'll need to wash it off and reapply it 2–3 times daily.

⚬ If your baby's mouth is affected, you can rinse it out with an infusion of *Calendula* flowers (see Appendix 5). *Thyme* is another herb which has antifungal and antimicrobial properties, but he may dislike the taste. Dip a clean, soft cloth in the infusion and swab the curds away from his tongue, gums and cheeks before and after each feed. You could also use a cotton bud.

⚬ You can try the same treatment with a solution of baking soda (1 teaspoon in a cup of boiled and cooled purified water). This must be made fresh each day.

⚬ You could coat your baby's mouth with yoghurt (the unsweetened, non-flavoured variety, preferably made from goat's milk). Dip your finger in the yoghurt, and let him suck it off, or use a cotton bud or cloth.

⚬ A good homoeopathic remedy for your baby is *Mercurius cyanatus*. Use in the 6c potency, just 5 drops under his tongue.

⚬ For your breasts you can use the same remedies you use for your baby's mouth, swabbing them with herbal infusions or coating them in yoghurt (a tasty accompaniment to the cabbage leaves we suggested earlier!)

⚬ You could try the mixture of vinegar and *Tea-tree* oil we suggest below for vaginal thrush on your breasts, but this must be washed off thoroughly before the next feed, as must herbs such as *Golden Seal*, *Barberry* and *Oregon Mountain Grape*, though these can be applied very successfully, even in quite severe cases. The more severe cases may need a stronger application, using the fluid extract of the herb rather than an infusion. These last three herbs contain an alkaloid, berberine, which is a powerful antimicrobial that is effective against bacteria, protozoa and fungi, but they should not be used internally while breastfeeding.

⚬ *Don't* use *Gentian Violet* for your baby's mouth or your breasts. This used to be a common treatment but although it is quite effective, it may be carcinogenic.

Be strict with your hygiene, wash your hands and breasts after each feed, and be careful how you contact infected areas.

Use any of the other remedies we have suggested for painful breasts or sore nipples, though these won't be effective unless you also deal with the yeast.

An excellent local vaginal treatment for candida is to use a *Tea-tree* based cream, or you could try acidophilus yoghurt (live culture) which can be very soothing. Treatment should be continued until symptoms have abated for several days, or you have a repeat vaginal swab which is clear.

You can douche with a mixture of 4 drops of *Tea-tree* oil and 2 tablespoons (50 mL) of white vinegar in two litres of warm water, or add it to a sitz-bath. Do not use cider vinegar (which is sometimes suggested) as it contains sugar. Your partner may also need treatment. He can dunk his penis in the same mixture. You may need to avoid having sex while treatment is carried out, since intercourse can cause the condition to flare up. (Strictly speaking, candida is an infestation, not an infection, and therefore cannot be 'caught'. However, it can spread to susceptible areas.)

A good herbal douche can be made from a mix of equal parts of *Golden Seal*, *Calendula* (both herbs are antifungal and antibacterial), *Uva Ursi* and *Witch Hazel* (astringent and antimicrobial). It can be used instead of, or added to, the *Tea-tree* and vinegar mix. Add a few drops of *Citrus Seed* extract.

If the vaginal infection is external rather than internal, you can sit in a basin or shallow bath and swish the mixture up into the vagina, or soak a tampon in the mixture and insert it, instead of using a douche. Never leave a tampon in place for longer than eight hours, as it could lead to toxic shock syndrome, and never use these treatments inside the vagina if you are, or could be, pregnant.

Aloe Vera gel can be very effective for vaginal thrush, especially if essential oil of *Marjoram* (an antifungal) is added. A clove of *Garlic* (unchipped and wrapped in gauze) can be inserted into the vagina. Leave a 'tail' on the gauze so you can pull it out. Don't use vinegar if you have any cuts or abrasions.

Treating systemic candida

If you find local treatments aren't sufficiently effective, the underlying problems must also be adequately addressed. First, an anti-candida diet must be rigorously followed. This diet excludes absolutely all refined carbohydrates and sugars, including alcohol, because they act as 'food' for the organism, which must be starved to be defeated. All products containing yeast (to which you may have become allergic) must also be strictly avoided, unless you are confident that they don't affect you adversely. The diet we have suggested in Chapter 5, if followed assid-uously, will address the problem, and you can assess your susceptibility to yeast products in the same way that we have outlined for other aller-gies earlier in this chapter. (There are many good books on candida and its treatment; see Recommended Reading.)

Next, you must not take antibiotics or the oral contraceptive pill, as these will make effective treatment very difficult to achieve. Antibiotics will destroy the good bacteria which help to keep the candida under control. Further, you'll need to undertake all the following measures.

- Kill the yeast: This can be achieved through drugs such as Nystatin, which can be used safely during lactation. However, you may prefer to use gentle, natural remedies such as *Garlic*, *Citrus Seed* extract, *Caprylic acid*, and herbs such as *Marjoram* and *Oregano*, both of which can be used in your cooking. A *Garlic* suppository (just a clove of garlic) can be inserted anally. *Garlic* contains *allicin*, which has strong antimicrobial properties, and possibly works by damaging the structure and integrity of the yeast cell wall. Some studies have shown it to be more potent than Nystatin, *Gentian Violet* and several other commonly used antifungal agents. *Citrus Seed* extract is a natural antimicrobial, but requires dilution as it is caustic. *Caprylic acid* is a fatty acid found in coconuts and palm oil, which has strong antifungal properties. As it is very readily absorbed in the gut, it will be most effective if it is enteric-coated to allow for gradual release. *Marjoram* and *Oregano* are effective antifungal herbs, which can be taken as infusions or fluid extracts for greater effectiveness. *Pau D'Arco* and *Calendula* are also very effective antifungal herbs, which have additional properties. *Calendula* is a bitter herb, which helps to restore gut function (see later), and *Pau D'Arco* supports the immune system.

❊ Starve the yeast: As we've already mentioned, you should eat no sugars (of any kind), no refined carbohydrates (white flours and grains), and no alcohol. (Not that you'd dream of eating or drinking any of these things anyway!) You should also avoid fruit for the first month of the treatment and then reintroduce it slowly. See Chapter 5 for more dietary advice.

❊ Stabilise blood sugar levels: This is necessary to help prevent sugar cravings, since sugar feeds the troublesome yeasts. Here we would use chromium, and bitter herbs such as *Dandelion Root, Agrimony* and *Fringetree. Gymnema* (a very bitter herb) can be used to quell sugar cravings as they arise, as it neutralises the sugar receptors on the tongue. Put 1 or 2 drops in a little water, and swill around the mouth.

❊ Avoid allergens: This list is likely to include yeast-containing and fermented foods and fungi, but any food to which you are allergic can compromise your immune system, irritate your gut and undermine recovery (see earlier in this chapter).

❊ Boost the immune system: You can do this with herbs such as *Echinacea, Siberian Ginseng* and *Cat's Claw*, and a full complement of nutrients, especially the B-complex vitamins and zinc. Candida sufferers are also often deficient in vitamin A, the omega-6 essential fatty acids, and magnesium.

❊ Repair the gut and re-establish gut flora: The average adult gut contains 1.5 kilos of over 400 strains of bacteria. These are beneficial bacteria which, in normal circumstances, keep the yeast under control. This healthy balance has to be restored, and you can achieve this with live *acidophilus, bifidus* and *bulgaris lactobacilli* (preferably in powder or tablet form, though live yoghurt is also useful as long as it contains no sugar or additives). Digestive enzymes (available in tablet form) can also assist healthy digestion, as can any of the 'bitter' herbs. These herbs stimulate the secretion of digestive juices in the stomach when they act on the bitter taste receptors in your mouth. Try herbs such as *Dandelion Root* and *St Mary's Thistle*. Plenty of fibre in your diet will also help to restore intestinal health, scouring the gut of harmful organisms. Eat lots of vegetables and, if there are problems with constipation, try taking *Psyllium* husks. *Slippery Elm* powder will coat the gut wall to reduce inflammation.

This treatment is likely to be required for two to three months in many cases before the problem is eradicated, though symptoms should die down quite quickly. Sometimes there can be an initial adverse reaction, when all symptoms temporarily flare up. This is called 'yeast die-off' as it's a result of the toxic yeast cells being killed and eliminated, and should be very temporary, especially if you're getting immune system support, and in most cases wellbeing will be quickly restored. In fact, as the candida infestation is brought under control, you should feel a lot healthier altogether as a chronic problem can be very debilitating. Don't worry if it takes a while to complete treatment; it's important to persevere.

A BITING BABY

Lots of new mothers think that it will be too difficult to breastfeed once their baby grows teeth. In fact, it's rarely a problem, and most babies don't bite. Your baby can't bite your nipple while he's sucking, so if you know he tends to bite, break the suction at the end of a feed as soon as he is satisfied and take him off your nipple. Also try not to feed him when he's not really hungry, he's restless, or has a snuffly nose. Good positioning is also important so the suction created when he's properly latched on isn't broken. Remember that your baby isn't malicious, and has no idea that biting can hurt you. Try not to react too sharply if it does happen, as you'll frighten him (yes we know he gave you a fright, too) and the feeding relationship will be disturbed. Teething should not need to be a reason for weaning—that should happen when your baby doesn't want or need to nurse any longer.

BREASTFEEDING IN PUBLIC

What a shame that we even need to discuss the issue of feeding your baby in public, or that women need any reassurance about the rights to do so. It's also interesting that breastfeeding in public is only an issue in supposedly advanced Western nations. In what we consider more backward parts of the world, and this includes countries where women are covered from head to toe in garments that reveal absolutely nothing, breastfeeding women are commonplace and raise no eyebrows at all. One day this might be the case in the West too, but it will only happen if women feed in public, not behind closed doors, and certainly not in public toilets! A breastfeeding mother is not an exhibitionist—she is simply doing the job that her breasts were designed for.

It will make it easier for you to feed discreetly if you always wear clothes that zip or button down the front, and if you feel a little uncomfortable at first a large shawl or a scarf can be draped so that nobody is really any the wiser. Always remember that nobody can ask you to leave or to go elsewhere to feed your baby, and we really believe that if you look confident and at ease, they are unlikely to do so. As we've already told you, Jan and Francesca fed their boys for a grand total of seventeen years, and not once in all their years of feeding anywhere and everywhere were they ever made to feel uncomfortable. Others might have been uncomfortable on their behalf, especially when small boys were unbuttoning their blouses, but that wasn't Jan or Francesca's problem.

In feeding your baby in public you are not only affirming the importance of what you are doing, but you are sending other women the message that it is fine for them to do the same.

11

Common problems for your breastfed baby

A DELAYED START TO BREASTFEEDING

There are very few reasons why your baby cannot feed just as soon after the birth as he wants to. Occasionally, a very premature baby or a baby requiring surgery may not be able to breastfeed (in which case you can express and store your milk), but even a Down Syndrome baby or one with a cleft palate can have a breastfeeding experience shortly after birth. When correctly established, early and frequent breastfeeding prevents lots of problems further down the track.

However, if you can't nurse your baby immediately, you can offer the expressed and stored colostrum from a dropper, cup or spoon when he is eventually able to take something by mouth. When he is ready to have the real thing, it can help him to get the hang of it if you start on a relatively empty breast. That way, he is less likely to be overwhelmed by the rush of milk. If he has to stay in hospital (in intensive care, for example), you'll need to stay close by so he can receive your expressed milk and breastfeed as soon as possible. Francesca's first son was in the 'premie' ward for three weeks, during which time she was there too, touching and holding him and encouraging him to suck.

THE SLEEPY BABY

If your baby is suffering from the effects of drugs that you received during labour, or if he was born prematurely, he may be very drowsy and this can make breastfeeding difficult to establish. A sleepy baby may also be diagnosed as suffering from low blood sugar. Whatever the reason for his drowsiness, it's important to get him interested in a feed just as often as you can and to nurse him before he cries. It also helps if your let-down reflex is already working when he comes to the breast; hot towels or compresses on your breast can get your milk flowing. It may also help if he's not too warmly dressed. Cold feet can keep him awake and feeding.

On the other hand, your baby may exhibit more interest in his surroundings in a situation that closely resembles his uterine environment. Keep the lighting down and take your baby into a warm bath with you. Let him lie on your chest and see if he will come to the breast that way. You should try to have as much skin-to-skin contact as possible. Try not to give in to the formula option—even though nursing a sleepy baby can be very discouraging, if you persevere your patience will be rewarded. Eventually he will start to wake up and exhibit real enthusiasm for your breast.

THE CRYING BABY

Your baby cries because he's trying to tell you something. He's not trying to be difficult; he's saying, 'Hey Mum, there's a problem here!' So when your baby cries, if he's not in your arms already pick him up straight away. He needs to know that you will respond. Then you need to find out what's wrong.

Babies truly only have a few needs. They need to be kept warm, dry and clean. They need to feel loved and wanted. They need to be fed. They need close physical contact, cuddles and caresses. They need to get enough sleep. They need to be comfortable and free from pain, and they need to learn and be stimulated. So you need to work out (with your baby's help) what the problem is and solve it for him if you can—because he can't. Putting a dummy in your baby's mouth does not solve any of his problems, it just starts him on a life of oral fixation. But let's look at what you can do to resolve some of those problems. You'll find that after you get used to your baby's cries you'll have a good idea of what his problem is as he'll use different cries for different situations.

Why is he crying?

Perhaps he's hungry

This is the most common reason for a baby to cry. But it's not the only reason. So don't assume that every time he cries he needs a feed and don't assume that you haven't got enough milk. We feel we've probably said enough about this already, but the worst thing you can do is give him a bottle. If he is hungry he'll suck your breast, and there's plenty of advice earlier in this book if you're really concerned that you don't have enough milk. If he is hungry and feeding isn't working, it's more likely to be due to poor positioning or attachment so go back to our advice on that in Chapter 3.

Perhaps he's feeling insecure

Your baby may need to feel like he did when he was in your womb, especially if he had a difficult birth. So pick him up and hold him. (We hope you never put him down.) Studies confirm what is fairly obvious: babies cry less if they are carried more. He may also need to nurse, regardless of whether he's hungry or you have any milk.

While you're holding him you can use tried and true soothers such as rocking and singing and stroking. A rocking chair is a wonderful investment, and wrapping yourself and your baby up in a big shawl (unless it's too hot) can calm you both to a gentle rhythm. You can also rock your baby to and fro while he's held over your shoulder, which is

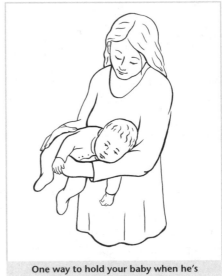

One way to hold your baby when he's upset or colicky

good for getting up wind, and many babies' preferred position. Another comfortable way to rock your baby is to lie him on his tummy along your arm, with his arms and legs dangling free and his head cradled by your elbow. This is especially helpful if he's colicky, or if you need a free hand.

Stroking his back and patting his bottom firmly but gently will probably come to you naturally, and you may be interested in learning baby or infant massage, to take this one step further. There are classes at which you and your partner can learn this ancient art. Lullabies have also been used from time immemorial; you may even remember some your mother sang to you. Don't be worried if you can't sing in tune, your baby will appreciate a gentle hum just as much.

Your baby may need extra reassurance if he's crying because he's been startled. It might have been bright lights or sudden or loud noises that scared him, or he may be over-stimulated by a lot of activity happening around him.

He may be bored, lonely or just plain irritable

Though over-stimulation can certainly make your baby tearful and jittery, another possible reason for his crying could be that he's under-stimulated. Babies crave new experiences, as long as they feel secure. Frustration and pent-up energy from a lack of activity or social inter-action can find expression in an angry roar that will stop you in your tracks. The same techniques of rocking, stroking and singing described above will work to engage your baby's attention and soothe him, but make sure you're not on edge yourself—he may be irritable because he's picking it up from you. Luckily it's difficult to remain uptight while you're swaying and chanting, but the longer you leave him to cry, the more upset he'll get, and the longer it will take to settle him. This, in turn, will be more likely to frustrate you, your frustration will be trans-mitted to him . . . and on it goes. We've already warned you against coffee and smoking; these can be a major cause of irritability in breastfed babies.

Maybe he's overtired

The late afternoon–early evening period is a notorious black spot for baby blues, as any negative emotion or pent-up energy from the day peaks for both of you. If possible, spend these hours with your baby, or at least in some activity involving him. If either of you is overtired or fatigued, this can make things worse. To prevent everything from unravelling, make sure that the quality of your breast milk is maintained throughout the day and into the late afternoon. As well as the advice we've already given you on nutrition, make sure you eat plenty of protein between 2 and 4 pm. Of particular importance are the essential fatty acids (see Chapter 5). These keep your milk rich and fatty and more satisfying.

Good quality, satisfying milk will also help if your baby is overtired at this time, but unable to get to sleep. If the techniques we've already suggested don't work, try taking him into a warm bath with you. Tip some infused *Chamomile* into the water, but don't use essential oils. If nothing else works, going for a walk or a drive has saved many a parent and child from reaching the end of their respective tethers.

He could be uncomfortable

A baby may cry to tell you he's too hot, too cold, too wet, too dirty or being squashed. Unless it's really warm, he should always have something on his feet. A lot of body heat is lost through the feet, and a baby's feet should not be cold. We see many babies, especially in Australia where people are often not used to coping with cold weather, who are well wrapped up against the cold, with a little pair of bare blue feet hanging out of their warm trousers. Likewise your baby's head should be covered if it's cold, especially if he hasn't much hair, since this is another exit point for body heat. On the other hand, don't overdress him—if he's too hot he'll become dehydrated, which is dangerous. Of course if your baby is nestled against your body, your body heat will keep him much warmer than booties and beanies.

If he's wet or dirty he needs his nappy changed, and you shouldn't leave this for too long or he'll get a sore bottom. Make sure his nappy, his clothing, his bedclothes and shawls are not too tight. Forget the old idea that a newborn needs swaddling so he feels he's still in the womb; he needs to be able to move around easily. And while you're at it, check for the apocryphal safety pin—sometimes they do come undone. (To avoid this problem, you may prefer to use one of the nifty gadgets which can replace safety pins, and have no sharp bits.)

Maybe he's in pain

Colic is a major problem, even for some breastfed babies, and we'll look at some of the causes and remedies for this condition later in this chapter. If you've eaten anything to which you or your baby are allergic, this can be a problem too (see more in Chapter 10).

There could be a more serious reason for your baby's crying; babies do get sick, and if he's in severe pain his cry could sound shrill and piercing, although, on the other hand, he may become extremely quiet. In either of these two extreme cases, if he doesn't respond to your attempts to soothe him you should seek medical attention. (Babies often react like this after vaccination and we'll give you our thoughts on that in our next book.)

Remedies for you and your crying baby

If your baby's crying is really getting to you, try some of the remedies we suggested in Chapter 4 for stress management. Flower essences such as *Red Chestnut*, which is for over-anxiety for another person, *Impatiens* for anxiety or frustration, *Walnut* for protection from outside influences and *Pine* for guilt might help you. Flower essences can be used for your baby too—a drop or two under his tongue is quite safe— and can have immediate and profound effects. If you're not sure which remedy is appropriate, try *Rescue Remedy* which is the stand-by for all emergencies.

Homoeopathic remedies can also work fast and effectively, and are similar to flower essences in that they are entirely non-toxic and safe for babies. Here are a few suggestions (see also Appendix 5):

- *Borax*—for babies who are easily startled, nervous (especially at night) or who dislike movement (even rocking)

- *Chamomilla*—for babies who are irritable or angry, and refuse to be comforted

- *Lycopodium*—for babies who are irritable during the day, though fine at night, and for those who are fearful of strangers or new situations

- *Pulsatilla*—for babies who are clingy, dependent and weepy

One dose of the 30c potency may be sufficient, though up to three doses can be required to stabilise your baby. Homoeopathic remedies need to be chosen with care, and you will get the best results by consulting a professional homoeopath.

After your baby is two months old, if feeding is well established you can give him a few sips of *Chamomile* tea, or use it in a vaporiser to create a calm atmosphere. Another very helpful remedy, especially for babies who had a difficult birth, is cranial osteopathy, which can realign the bones in the skull that may have been pushed out of alignment during the birth.

THE BABY WHO WON'T SETTLE TO FEED

If your baby won't settle down to feed, you need first of all to be sure he's hungry. He can't tell you if he isn't, he can only refuse the breast. Check all those things we talked about in Chapter 3: make sure his nose is clear of your breast, that you are both positioned comfortably and that he's attached well, with the whole areola in his mouth. In Chapter 10 we gave advice on dealing with milk that is too profuse or coming out too fast. You could also think back to any unusual food you may have eaten in the last little while, as babies can dislike certain tastes, as well as having sensitivities or allergies.

It's also possible, if your cycle has returned and you're currently ovulating or menstruating, that the changing hormones may have affected the taste of your milk and caused him to be less eager to suckle. If so, don't worry, the effect is temporary and normal feeding will resume soon. A good homoeopathic remedy for a baby who's reluctant to feed, even though your milk is sufficient, is *Calc carb*. Lastly, check your mood—maybe you're the one who is unsettled.

THE BABY WHO NEEDS TREATMENT

If your baby needs treatment, the best and easiest way to achieve this is for you to take the remedy so he will get an appropriately smaller dose through your milk. In the case of acupressure or reflexology, his body will respond to pressure on the same points as those recommended for adults. This treatment can be incorporated into a baby massage.

THE SNUFFLY BABY

If your baby has nasal congestion, it's going to be difficult for him to feed. If he had mucus removed from his nose or throat after birth, this may have irritated his mucous membranes causing them to produce extra mucus, or he may have contracted a cold or upper respiratory tract infection (though this is less likely if he's breastfed).

If he can't breathe through his nose, he'll try to breathe through his mouth. In order to do so, he'll push the breast slightly out of his mouth, which will result in poor attachment and insufficient flow of milk. So he'll be hungry, but unable to satisfy his needs, and he'll be unsettled and want to feed often. In this case, you may need to express some milk and give it to him from a spoon, dropper or cup.

If the congestion isn't severe, you can use your breast milk to clear your baby's nose. While he's sucking on your finger, drip about 10 drops of expressed milk into each nostril. It will run down into his throat and be swallowed quite easily, though if it makes him cough, you should stop. Then clear his nose with a twist of tissue. If you take extra *Garlic* or some *Fenugreek* tea, this may help to clear his mucosa, and *Echinacea* will transfer through the milk to fight any infection.

JAUNDICE

Bilirubin is the yellow pigment responsible for the suntanned appearance of a jaundiced baby. It is formed when the haem portion of red blood cells breaks down. In utero, your placenta acts as a filter for these breakdown products, but after birth your baby's liver has to take over the task. During the early weeks of life there is a rapid turnover of red blood cells and your baby's mechanisms for excretion can't quite keep pace.

It has always been the practice to treat jaundice aggressively (with abundant fluids and phototherapy lights) because too much bilirubin can lead to brain damage. However it now appears that the presence of some bilirubin may be beneficial. Bilirubin is an antioxidant and newborns are deficient in these vitally important substances. It seems that nature has taken a waste product and converted it into a protective agent. But when does enough become too much?

Feeding your baby soon after birth clears meconium from your baby's gut and leads to lowered bilirubin levels. If you then feed your baby every two hours the bilirubin levels should have halved by day 3. Studies have shown that the optimal frequency to achieve the lowest bilirubin levels is 11 feeds in 24 hours. While conventional treatment involves abundant fluids, giving water exacerbates jaundice, so make sure that the only fluid your jaundiced baby receives is from your breast. Also avoid vitamin K injections for your baby—these increase the risk of jaundice. Oral administration of vitamin K causes fewer problems. (See *Healthy Body, Better Birthing* for more information on vitamin K.)

There are also a few natural remedies you can try.

- Take liver herbs—*Dandelion Root, St Mary's Thistle* or *Schisandra*—as teas or fluid extracts. Your baby will get his dose through your breast milk.

- In severe cases, and with professional supervision, *Dandelion Root, St Mary's Thistle* or *Schisandra* can be given directly to your baby. Place a few drops under his tongue every four hours, or rub a few drops on your nipple before feeds. Alternatively, you could try the remedies known as 'homoeobotanicals'. These are herbs rendered potent in the manner of a homoeopathic remedy which can be given in very small doses. This treatment should only be continued for a few days or until the condition improves.

- Put a few drops of the homoeopathic remedy *Aconite* (in 200c potency) on your nipples before each feed. This should only be done for a single day.

- The tissue salt *Nat Sulph* can be given indirectly to your baby via your breast milk. Take 8 pilules three times daily, or if using the celloids (in which case the remedy is called 'SS') take 2 tablets 3 times daily.

- Exposing your baby to warm sunlight, avoiding the hottest part of the day, can achieve the same effect as phototherapy lights in hospitals.

- Place one red and one blue veil over your baby's sleeping place to filter the sunlight and create a violet light. This is another low-tech alternative to the ultraviolet lamps that are used in hospitals. It avoids the problem of electromagnetic fields surrounding your child.

≈ Keep breastfeeding, even if you are still only producing colostrum.

Occasionally, jaundice may not respond to these measures. In that case you should seek medical advice.

COLIC

There's still a lot of mystery surrounding colic and there's even some thought that there's really no such thing. Try telling that to a mother with a colicky baby and you risk serious derision, but it's interesting to observe babies in traditional cultures—there colic certainly doesn't seem to be the problem that it is for women and babies in Western society.

Essentially, colic is due to spasm in your baby's intestinal muscle causing abdominal cramp, a bit like severe indigestion. Babies who suffer from colic have been found to have high levels of motilin, a gut hormone that modulates gastrointestinal motility, but nobody really knows why this occurs. It may be that there is no single cause of colic, but several. These include the possibility that the baby's gut may be immature with inefficient peristalsis (the waving motion which helps food pass along the intestine) or insufficient gut flora. The baby may suffer from heartburn or may have a bowel infection. Babies who have suffered birth trauma or whose mothers suffered severe stress or illness during pregnancy or birth seem to be more prone to colic, as do babies who are overstimulated or excited when they feed.

More commonplace causes of colic include overfeeding and swallowing air, both of which can result from the milk flowing too fast. Conversely, some babies display colicky symptoms when they are hungry, especially when going through a growth spurt. Other causes may include feeding with a cold tummy (so make sure your baby is warm), insufficient burping and feeding only the foremilk, which is high in lactose. Many cases seem to be the result of the mother's diet. We'll look at remedies for all of these in a moment, but don't be too concerned. Apart from the distress caused to both you and your baby, there's seldom anything seriously wrong. However, colic can make your breastfeeding experience less than perfect.

Colic usually begins when your baby is between 1–4 weeks of age, and rarely continues beyond 3–4 months. It's often worse at the same time each day, most usually the early evening, and can be brief or go on for hours. Your baby is likely to have a loud, persistent, intense and piercing cry. Try not to get too anxious about this, as it could make him worse. He may also have a red face, or a pale face with a bluish tinge on his upper lip. He's likely to pull his knees up to his tummy, or stretch his legs out rigidly and arch his head and body backwards. He may move his arms vigorously, with his fists clenched. His tummy may be tense and distended, and could be accompanied by burping, flatulence or rumbling noises. Try to remind yourself that he is unlikely to be ill, and that he will grow out of it.

Hopefully you will be able to bring relief through some of the following suggestions. However, if the screaming continues for hours on end, or is accompanied by fever, persistent vomiting, diarrhoea, constipation or lack of urine, you should seek medical help.

- See if your baby needs burping. Put him up against your shoulder and gently pat his back. Burping is not always necessary after a feed, and thumping his back should be avoided. You may find it easier to put him over your knee and rub his back, or lie him along your arm as we suggested earlier. If he brings up a little milk, he may be hungry again and need another feed. If you carry your baby close or in a sling, the movement will bring up excess air naturally, and you may not need to make a special effort to burp him. Following our suggestions for managing too much milk or milk that flows too fast (see Chapter 10) will help to stop him swallowing air when he feeds. Also feed him often so he doesn't get desperately hungry and gulp.

- All the remedies we've suggested for calming a crying baby— rocking, car rides, warm baths with herbal infusions etc—are relevant now, for you as well as him.

- Warmth can help. A warm bath, or a warm hot-water bottle or a nappy or towel soaked in warm water and placed on his tummy can be very soothing. An infusion of *Chamomile*, *Lavender* or *Lemon Balm* can be added to the bath or the water in which you soak the nappy.

- Massaging your baby can soothe him and ease the pain. Gently rub his tummy in a clockwise direction, following the path of the large intestine. Also rub his back, and bend his knees and push them gently into his tummy. This may release some gas. He may also get relief if you move his legs in a bicycling action. Although you need to be very careful using essential oils on new babies, when you're massaging you could try adding 2 drops of *Fennel*, *Dill*, *Chamomile* or *Lavender* essential oil to 30 mL of an almond oil base. Massaging your baby's feet and hands can also help, as you will be stimulating the reflex points for his large and small intestines and his stomach.

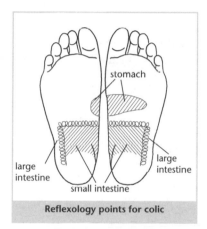

Reflexology points for colic

A baby fed from both breasts at each feed may receive only the foremilk that is high in lactose. Difficulty digesting the lactose can give your baby colic. Feed from one breast only at each feed, or at least make sure the first breast is drained fully before you move on to the second. This makes sure your baby gets the fatty hindmilk.

Eat a diet that has plenty of protein and avoid refined carbohydrates; this also keeps lactose levels down. See Chapter 5 for more on a healthy diet.

Certain foods that you eat, particularly dairy foods, wheat, eggs, citrus fruits, peanuts and the brassica family (cabbage, cauliflower, brussel sprouts, broccoli, turnips, radishes and kale) can cause colic in your baby. Also take care with nuts, strawberries, peaches, plums, pineapple, grapes, garlic, onions, green peppers, legumes, beans and fried or spicy foods. We've already warned you against alcohol and sugar and food and drinks containing caffeine. If this list seems daunting, don't be too concerned. Only some babies react to each food, though you'll also need to be aware of foods to which you are allergic (see Chapter 10 for more on this). In one study a diet free of wheat and dairy foods was found to be effective in relieving 80 per cent of colic cases.

Make sure you're getting appropriate nutritional supplementation (see Chapter 5).

Avoid laxatives which can irritate your baby as they pass through your milk. Too much fruit can also have this effect. (This includes dried fruit.)

You can use your milk as a channel for helpful remedies. Herbal infusions that you drink will transfer through the milk to your baby in appropriately smaller concentration. (See Appendix 5 for how to make an infusion.) Helpful herbs include:
- *Chamomile* flowers, *Fennel* seeds, *Dill* seeds, *Caraway* seeds, *Cumin* seeds and *Aniseed* seeds (crack the seeds first) to soothe the gut
- *Ginger*, *Cloves*, *Cinnamon Bark* to dispel gas
- *Wild Yam* and *Cramp Bark* for cramping
- *Catnip* (which is also a smooth muscle relaxant and relieves flatulence), *Lemon Balm*, *Lavender* and *Chamomile* for the sedative effect.

You can give herbal infusions directly to your baby using an eye-dropper, spoon or cup. Make sure you use purified water and strain the tea well. If your baby is less than six months old, 5 mL 2–3 times daily may be enough. If he is between 6 and 12 months increase this to 10 mL; after he is 12 months try 20–30 mL.

Gripe Water is a popular traditional remedy sold through pharmacies, which contains *Fennel* and *Dill*, but unfortunately it is also full of sugar.

Slippery Elm is an excellent remedy for an irritated gut if your baby is over 3 months old. Half a teaspoon can be mixed with purified boiled water and a little maple syrup to form gruel (like a slippery form of porridge). Feed it to your baby with a spoon. Although we don't normally recommend sweeteners, we don't think he's likely to accept this mixture without something to alleviate the less than pleasant taste. Make sure you use genuine maple syrup, not the chemically-flavoured topping. Honey should not be used as a sweetener for children under 12 months as, although it has antiseptic qualities, it may contain micro-organisms with which their less developed immune systems may not be able to cope. Half a teaspoon of a protein powder which is made from whey can be mixed in as well. This contains no casein or lactose, but is full of antibodies like those in colostrum. If this is not available, a mixture of acidophilus and bifidus lactobacilli in powder form can be used instead.

* Homoeopathic remedies include *Dioscorea* if your baby's arching his back, *Colocynthis* if he's bent double and improves with firm pressure on his tummy, *Chamomilla* if he's restless, irritable and cranky, teething, or has one red and one pale cheek, *Carbo vegetabilis* if he's burping or has flatulence, *Mag phos* if warmth and gentle pressure on his tummy is helpful, and *Bryonia* if he's irritable and made worse by movement or jarring. Homoeopathic remedies are non-toxic to your baby, and can easily be administered as drops under his tongue (the dose is 5 drops every 2 hours for babies and toddlers). Use the 12c potency (30c for *Chamomilla*) or, better still, be guided by a homoeopath.

* Tissue salts can be obtained as pilules which dissolve under the tongue. For very young babies they should be dissolved first in water and administered with a dropper. *Mag phos* (MP) and *Nat sulph* (SS) can be given before a feed, and *Nat phos* (SP) is helpful for flatulence and gas. The dose is 1 pilule for babies up to 1 month, 2 pilules for infants aged 1–6 months, and 4 pilules for children 6 months–2 years, to be given every 1–2 hours, depending on the severity of the symptoms. If using normal-sized tablets (celloids), use ⅛ tablet for babies up to 1 month, ¼ tablet for infants aged 1–6 months and ½ tablet for children 6 months–2 years.

> *Rescue Remedy* and other flower essences to help emotional distress can be used for both you and your baby with no fear of reaction. Two drops for him and 6 for you every few hours, will help to calm you both and ease trauma.

> Cranial osteopathy can quite magically resolve colic in some babies, especially those who had a difficult birth.

> Acupuncture can be performed on quite tiny babies safely. Get your acupuncturist to show you points you can include in your baby massage.

DIARRHOEA

Breastfed babies normally have fairly loose, pasty stools, so it's important not to frighten yourself into thinking your baby has diarrhoea when he doesn't. What you need to watch for is a marked change in the consistency, appearance or smell of his poo, and associated symptoms such as fever, vomiting, loss of appetite, tummy cramps, weakness, shivering or obvious upset. Abnormal stools may contain mucus or little flecks of blood, be explosive, green, darker or paler than usual and a lot more watery. The smell may be sour or offensive.

Most cases of infant diarrhoea will resolve within 24 hours, and babies who are receiving nothing but breast milk seldom have a gastric infection. Although the cause of diarrhoea in breastfed babies may be bacterial, viral or parasitic, it is more often due to a change in your diet; for example, eating too much fruit or fat. (Fruit juice is a common cause of diarrhoea in babies who are not exclusively breastfed.) Any substance that is toxic or to which your baby has an allergy or sensitivity could also be a cause, as could antibiotics. Essentially your baby has diarrhoea because his body is trying to get rid of an irritating, toxic or infectious substance, though it can also be triggered by overstimulation or anxiety.

Dehydration is the major concern, especially if the diarrhoea is frequent and persists. You will need to breastfeed your baby frequently, and it's important that he has no solid food. If he's not interested in the breast (unlikely, especially as it will comfort him) or if the diarrhoea persists for more than a day, it's possible he may need extra water. He'll be more able to absorb the water if it has a *very* small amount of fruit juice added to it. You can add a quarter of a cup of fresh orange or lemon juice or a teaspoon of maple syrup (the genuine variety—but not honey if your baby's under one year old) to a litre of purified boiled water, and give small amounts hourly through a dropper, spoon or cup. You can also express your milk to give this way. Always seek advice, but don't let anyone persuade you to stop breastfeeding. If this is suggested, seek another opinion. Talk to the Australian Breastfeeding Association or a lactation expert as well as your doctor. You will need to seek medical advice if the diarrhoea is accompanied by any of these symptoms:

- fever
- fast pulse
- dehydration (dry tongue and mouth)
- loose skin or sudden weight loss (a sign of dehydration)
- sunken fontanelle or eyes (a sign of dehydration)
- sparse, dark or infrequent urine (a sign of dehydration)
- vomiting for more than 4 hours
- lack of appetite or poor feeding
- lethargy or drowsiness.

You should also consult a doctor if the diarrhoea persists.

If antibiotics are used or if they have caused the diarrhoea your baby will need some live yoghurt or a paste of half a teaspoon of acidophilus and bifidus lactobacilli powder mixed with a little genuine maple syrup and purified boiled water.

It's important to check your diet for problematic foods, especially any food which is new to your baby (see the section on colic and Chapter 10 for more on this). You'll also need to watch that your baby's bottom doesn't get sore. Make sure it's kept as dry and clean as possible by wiping it after each motion with moistened cotton wool and gently patting it dry. Zinc or *Calendula* cream or ointment will help to reduce soreness and irritation. Here are some other helpful remedies.

- Massaging your baby's tummy may help him, especially if the diarrhoea is accompanied by cramps. See the section on colic for how to do this, and also for helpful points to rub on his feet.

- Although you need to be very careful using essential oils on new babies, 1–2 drops of *Lavender* oil in 30 mL of almond oil may be used when you are massaging his tummy. If he's over a year old, you can add *Geranium* and *Peppermint* in the same amounts.

❧ Homoeopathic remedies are safe, non-toxic and powerful. Remedies for diarrhoea include:
- *Aconite* if the diarrhoea occurs after exposure to cold wind
- *Arsenicum album* if your baby has frequent, dark, scalding or putrid smelling motions; is restless, thirsty or weak; vomits immediately after feeding or if even water is vomited up. If relief is not prompt, it's time to get medical help. *Arsenicum album* is also useful if you suspect the cause of diarrhoea is too much fruit or fruit juice.
- *Chamomile* if the stools are greenish and slimy, especially during teething
- *Colocynthis* if the diarrhoea is accompanied by severe cramping or there's an explosive rush after feeding
- *Dulcamara* if the diarrhoea occurs after your baby has caught cold in damp weather or been exposed to damp conditions, or if his stool is yellow and watery and he has abdominal pain
- *Nux vomica* if the diarrhoea is a result of overfeeding, or your baby's straining to pass a small amount of watery poo at each attempt
- *Podophyllum* if his poo is watery and explosive, and comes straight after feeding or bathing, especially early in the morning

See the section on colic for dosage guidelines. In acute situations you can increase the frequency of the dose to every half hour.

❧ Herbal remedies can be given through the breast milk as infusions, tinctures or extracts or given directly as infusions. See the section on colic for dosage guidelines. Useful herbs include *Raspberry* and *Meadowsweet*, which are both traditionally used for children's diarrhoea, while *Marshmallow Root* and *Chamomile* will both soothe your baby's tummy, and *Chamomile* will also help to calm him if he's irritable or upset, as will *Lemon Balm*. *Slippery Elm* given as gruel can help, as we suggested for colic.

❧ Tissue salts can be very effective and fast-acting. They are very gentle remedies which are safe for your baby. See the section on colic for dosage guidelines for these salts:

- *Ferrum phos* (IP) if there is fever or infection
- *Kali mur* (PC) if there is vomiting
- *Kali phos* (PP) if there is dehydration
- *Nat phos* (SP) if there are sour, acid stools
- *Nat sulph* (SS) if there is an offensive odour
- *Mag phos* (MP) if there is bloating

CONSTIPATION

Breastfed babies often don't have a bowel motion every day. You only need to be concerned if your baby's stool is too hard, dry, accompanied by straining or if there are other symptoms such as pain, bloating, vomiting or loss of appetite.

Constipation is usually the result of dietary considerations, either what you are eating and passing on through the milk, or what your baby is eating if he's started on solids. Too much meat or too many eggs can cause constipation, as can dairy foods, refined flour products or any food to which you or he are allergic or sensitive. Bananas are often used as a first baby food and can cause constipation if they are unripe. Beware of bananas if the skin doesn't peel easily or if they are green; it's better for your baby if the skin has started to go black.

Make sure your diet is free of problem foods, and that you're eating plenty of vegetables, and some fruit. You can increase the amount of fruit to encourage softer motions for your baby. Also make sure you're both getting plenty of fluid; your breast milk will be enough for your baby if he's feeding frequently. Vitamin C and magnesium will be helpful nutritional supplements for you to take. You can also use the same gruel of *Slippery Elm* and lactobacilli that we suggested for diarrhoea. As these remedies help to soothe and coat the gut, they are appropriate for treating conditions that result in motions that are too hard or infrequent as well as those that cause loose watery stools. Powdered *Psyllium* husks, which are a good bulking agent, can be added to the gruel for constipated babies. Similarly, the massage over the abdomen and on foot reflex points that we described for colic and diarrhoea can also be used for constipation.

Avoid laxatives, even if they are natural or herbal, as they are irritating to the gut and habit-forming. However, some natural remedies may help. (See the section on colic for dosages.)

⚸ Herbs to try include *Dandelion Root*, *Fennel Seed* and *Ginger*.
Chamomile and *Cramp Bark* will help if there is spasm or
cramping, and *Marshmallow Root* and *Slippery Elm* will help to
soften the stool. Tissue salts that may help are *Nat sulph* (SS) and
Mag phos (MP).

⚸ You may find your baby gets relief if treated with these
homoeopathic remedies:
  ● *Alumina* if his stool is hard, or evacuation is painful even though
    his stool is soft. *Alumina* also helps if there are very few motions
  ● *Bryonia* if your baby's faeces are large, hard, dry and very dark
  ● *Graphites* if your baby has no urge to defecate, then after days
    of no stool has one made up of round balls with mucus which are
    painful to pass
  ● *Nat mur* if the faeces resemble hard pellets, or the stool is hard
    and crumbly, accompanied by blood and a sore bottom
  ● *Nux vomica* if your baby has constant urging to defecate, but no
    faeces are passed
  ● *Silica* if his stool starts to come, then retreats. Also use *Silica* if
    there is mucus present in his stool, or he has a sore anus
  ● *Taraxacum* if your baby has no appetite or is bloated. Also use
    Taraxacum if his tongue has a white coating under which there
    are dark red and sensitive patches

⚸ Although you need to take care with essential oils, *Lavender* can
be used in the massage oil for your baby's tummy, as for diarrhoea.
If he is over three years old you can add *Rosemary* and *Marjoram*.

⚸ An extra point to use when massaging your baby's hands is
Colon 4, which you'll find in the apex of the 'V' formed by the
bones of his index finger and his thumb, on the back of his hand.
Another useful point is *Triple Heater 6* which is on his forearm
between the two bones, four of his finger-widths from the bend of
his wrist, on the outer side. Use a clockwise motion when stimulating these points.

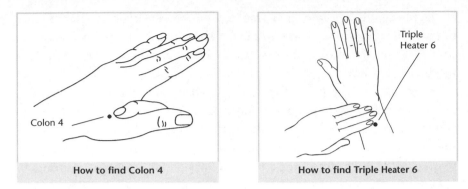

| How to find Colon 4 | How to find Triple Heater 6 |

REFLUX AND VOMITING

It is normal for your baby to bring up some of his milk after feeding, but it may cause you concern if it becomes too frequent or seems to cause him distress. It's called 'posseting' when he throws up small amounts of his feed, usually as a result of overfeeding. This can happen simply because he goes on feeding for comfort after he's full. Although this is nothing to worry about (apart from having to wash your clothes more often or go around with permanent milk stains), you may find some help in the 'Too much milk' section of the previous chapter. If your baby's putting on weight, urinating frequently and seems well he's probably fine.

However, vomiting may have a more serious cause such as the rejection of toxins, or bacterial or other infection. Allergy, parasites (worms), travel sickness and shock may also cause vomiting. If the vomiting is accompanied by the following symptoms, you should seek medical attention:

- frequent vomiting with fever (it may be food poisoning)
- acute diarrhoea
- dehydration
- abnormal drowsiness
- refusing to feed
- the vomit is green or yellow
- the vomit continues for more than 2 hours
- vomiting in large amounts occurs after every feed, and your baby seems distressed
- the vomiting is associated with a head injury, stiff neck or severe abdominal pain

Projectile vomiting in the early weeks, when the entire stomach contents are hurled violently for some distance, can be caused by pyloric stenosis; that is when the exit from the stomach is too narrow. This requires medical attention.

Dehydration is a major concern if vomiting is persistent or frequent and large amounts of milk are brought up, or if it's accompanied by diarrhoea. Make sure your baby's getting plenty of fluids (see the section on diarrhoea for more on this) and don't stop breastfeeding. You may need to give fluids, including breast milk, in very small, frequent amounts to prevent further vomiting. Again, as with diarrhoea, you need to look at your diet for possible causes such as allergens, too much fatty food etc. Vitamin B6 can help nausea, and you can try taking 100 mg extra daily. Don't exceed this dose, and don't continue if you feel your milk supply diminishes as vitamin B6 can affect the production of prolactin.

Some babies have a weakness associated with the small valves at the top of their stomachs, which may be immature when they are little. This can cause reflux (sometimes called oesophageal reflux) either during or after a feed, as they can't keep the breast milk in their stomach. If the regurgitated milk isn't vomited out it can cause severe discomfort, as the contents of the stomach spill back into the oesophagus, resulting in heartburn, inflammation, or even ulceration. This can be worsened if the baby overfeeds, seeking relief in the antacid effect of the milk. Symptoms include frequent posseting, irritability during or after feeds, coughing or choking during feeds and frequent or irregular feeding which can result in excessive weight gain. If you think your baby is experiencing reflux, seek medical advice, though some of the following remedies may bring some relief.

- For persistent vomiting try a hot pack on your baby's tummy. (Heat applied to the stomach reduces spasms.) A hot-water bottle, well covered with a cloth nappy, may help, or you can try a hot salt pack. Heat a cup of sea salt in a pan for 5 minutes and pour it into a cloth container such as a pillowcase which you then fold until it's the size of your baby's tummy. Wrap it well in a cloth nappy as salt gets very hot.

- The herb that is most generally used for vomiting or nausea is *Ginger*, but *Aniseed*, *Chamomile*, *Cinnamon*, *Cloves*, *Fennel* seeds and *Raspberry* have also been found to help. *Meadowsweet* and

Lemon Balm have a particularly soothing effect on the stomach. See the section on colic for dosage guidelines.

✳ *Slippery Elm* can be used as for diarrhoea, though you may find your baby can't tolerate it if he's feeling too nauseated.

✳ You can massage your baby's tummy to give him some relief (see the section on diarrhoea for more on this). If he's over 12 months old, you can add a few drops of *Peppermint* oil to some almond oil to make this more effective, or sprinkle it on a cloth for him to inhale. If he's over 3 years you can also use *Sandalwood* oil.

✳ Homoeopathic remedies are, again, easy to use and effective. Try these:
  * *Aconite* if he's vomiting up his whole feed immediately and seems chilled. Also if he vomits as a result of spoilt food or too much fruit, or if he's vomiting as a result of being frightened or startled.
  * *Aethusa cynapium* if the milk comes straight up again as thick, acid clots, and the vomiting is followed by weakness and sleepiness
  * *Bryonia* if he vomits as a result of too much rich or fatty food, or if he is irritable
  * *Ipecacuanha* if vomiting is persistent after eating, especially if his tongue is clean
  * *Nux vomica* if he vomits after too much rich or different food

✳ There are two acupressure points you can stimulate on your baby to help nausea or vomiting. One is *Pericardium 6* which you can

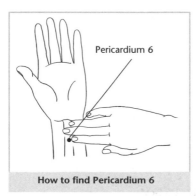

How to find Pericardium 6

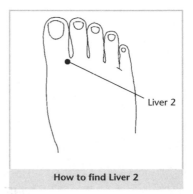

How to find Liver 2

find three of his finger-widths up the inside of his arm from his wrist crease, between the two tendons (the third finger finds the spot). The other is *Liver 2* which you can find between the large and second toes, slightly up from the edge of the web and closer to his big toe.

ORAL THRUSH

If your baby has a coating on his tongue and inner cheeks which is clottier than the residue of milk after a feed and is not easily scraped off, he may be suffering from oral thrush. If so, he may also have a red flaky rash on his bottom, in the crease of his neck and on his thighs and in his armpits. If you have a daughter, she may have white curds in her labial folds.

Thrush, also known as candida, can transfer to your breast and create major problems with breastfeeding, as well as causing discomfort to your baby. See Chapter 10 for treatments for both of you—treating yourself or your baby alone may not be sufficient.

Although the natural remedies we've suggested in the last two chapters are effective and safe, we sincerely hope that you never have to use them.

Those of you who have read our previous books, and followed our recommendations before and during pregnancy, are much less likely to experience any problems during breastfeeding.

Even if you've only come to the 'Natural Way' after the birth of your baby, you'll be less likely to need remedies if you follow our suggestions earlier in this book on ways to make breastfeeding a 'better' experience.

Epilogue

Make the most of the time you're breastfeeding. Marvel at the ease and simplicity of it all, revel in the closeness and the intimacy and enjoy it for just as long as your baby wants it. By the time he's ready to move away from the comfort of your breast you'll be ready for our next book, *The Natural Way to Raise a Better Baby*.

In the meantime we hope that when you breastfeed in the manner we've proposed, you will always be completely at ease with following your child's personal agenda through his early years. We hope our endorsement of breastfeeding wherever, whenever and for as long as your baby needs it, and our encouragement to 'follow your child' will ensure that there are lots of truly better babies. It will be these truly better babies who will grow into well-adjusted, highly functional adults, and it will be these adults who will be best able to deal with the challenges of the new millenium. It is these same adults who will, in turn, be able to breastfeed and successfully nurture better babies of their own, or wholeheartedly support their partners in their mothering during this vitally important period of their children's early years.

Safety of medical drugs during breastfeeding

Aciclovir
Topical treatment for herpes is not secreted into breast milk, but should be washed off nipples before breastfeeding.

Alcohol
AVOID: see Chapter 6

Antibiotics
Penicillin and *cephalosporin* groups are safe, (including *amoxicillin*).
AVOID: *chloramphenicol, metronidazole, nalidixic acid, tetracyclines*

Antidepressants
Surprisingly little is passed into the milk but watch for drowsiness.
AVOID: *fluoxetine (Prozac), doxepin, lithium, MAO inhibitors*

Anti-epileptics
Phenytoin and *sodium valproate* are most commonly used, but monitor baby for sedation.

Antifungals
Nystatin (for thrush, candida) is unlikely to be absorbed.
AVOID: *miconazole*

Antihistamines
May cause drowsiness.
AVOID: Chronic use, long-acting products, *astemizole, terfenadine*

Antihypertensives
Methyldopa, propranolol, nifedipine and *minoxidil* are best.
AVOID: ACE inhibitors

Antimalarials
Small amounts enter breast milk and some babies may become jumpy.

Asthma drugs
Sodium cromoglycate (Intal) is safe. *Ventolin* and *Bricanyl* inhalers cause no reported ill effects. *Steroids* via inhaler do not affect the baby. (See also **Steroids, oral dose**.)

Caffeine
AVOID: see Chapter 6

Cough medicines
May cause drowsiness if they contain antihistamines.
AVOID: products containing *iodine* and *guaiphenesin*

Diuretics
All reduce milk supply.
AVOID

Hexachlorophene
Transferred to milk through your skin.
AVOID and do not use on the baby's skin either

Insulin
Not secreted into milk.

Laxatives
Bulking agents are not absorbed from your gut so are unlikely to affect the baby.
AVOID: Aperients (which stimulate the gut)

Methotrexate
AVOID

Migraine drugs
These are toxic if used long-term or in high doses.

Oral contraceptives
AVOID: see Chapter 9

Painkillers
Use *paracetamol* or *ibuprofen*. *Diclofenac* (*Voltaren*) given after a Caesarean, does not enter breast milk in harmful amounts.
AVOID: *aspirin, morphine, pethidine* and *codeine* (in first 2 weeks)

Radioactive iodine
Present in breast milk for up to 96 hours. You must express milk in advance and discard milk for 16 days after tests are completed.

Radiopaque agents
Do not enter breast milk.

Recreational drugs
AVOID: see Chapter 6

Sedatives and hypnotics
Express milk in advance and discard milk while taking drug for short term.

Steroids, oral dose
Express milk in advance and discard milk while taking drug over short term.
Prednisolone is safe in low doses.

Tamoxifen
If you need to take this anti-cancer drug you should not breastfeed.

Thyroid drugs
Propylthiouracil for over-active thyroid enters breast milk and baby will need monitoring. *Thyroxine* and *liothyronine* for under-active thyroid are safe, but monitoring is required.

Tranquillisers
May cause drowsiness and problems with breastfeeding. *Oxazepam* (in low doses) is preferable to *diazepam* (*Valium*). Take special care if using *chlorpromazine* (*Largactil*) or *haloperidol* (*Serenace*).

APPENDIX 2

Safety of herbal remedies during breastfeeding

We've included here a list of herbs that we know are contraindicated during breastfeeding, or need to be used with caution. We've also included a list of commonly used herbs (for general health conditions) which are safe to take. For any others, consult a naturopath or herbalist. Many herbal constituents are excreted in breast milk and are thus transmitted from mother to baby while nursing, though usually in very reduced amounts, between 1 and 10 per cent. While this may usefully constitute a method for treating the baby (by having the mother ingest the remedy), it also means you need to take care. Culinary use is usually safe (but avoid *Sage* as it dries up your milk). Note that herbal teas must also be checked for suitability.

Any person may have an allergic reaction to a plant. Exclude any plants you know you are allergic to. If your baby shows distress after using any remedy, herbal or otherwise, discontinue its use and seek professional advice.

COMMONLY USED HERBS WHICH ARE SAFE TO USE WHILE BREASTFEEDING

Alfalfa	useful for all acidic conditions
Black Haw	useful for spasm or cramping
Burdock	useful for skin and gut problems
Calendula	useful for all skin problems
Catnip	useful for anxiety or sleeplessness
Chamomile	useful for all stress and gastrointestinal conditions
Cleavers	useful for lymphatic detoxification
Corn Silk	useful for urinary tract problems
Cramp Bark	useful for spasm or cramping
Dandelion Leaf	useful for fluid retention
Dandelion Root	useful for the liver and digestion
Dill Seed	useful for digestion, flatulence
Dong Quai	useful for problems of the reproductive system
Echinacea	useful for all infections
Fennel	useful for flatulence and indigestion
Fenugreek	useful for all catarrhal conditions
Ginkgo	useful for all circulatory and mental problems
Garlic	useful for all infections
Hops	useful for nervous disorders, insomnia
Lavender	useful for stress, headaches
Lemon Balm	useful for depression, stress
Marshmallow Root	useful for irritation of gut or urinary tract
Nettle	useful for urinary tract problems
Oats	useful for depression, nervous stress
Raspberry	useful for uterine problems, diarrhoea
Skullcap	useful for insomnia, anxiety, stress
Slippery Elm	useful for irritated gut, constipation
St Mary's Thistle	useful for all liver conditions
Witch Hazel	useful for bleeding or discharge
Withania	useful for fatigue, stress
Culinary herbs	excluding *Sage*

Herbs that we have used elsewhere in the book as remedies for you or your baby are all known to be safe.

HERBS WHICH SHOULD BE USED WITH CAUTION WHILE BREASTFEEDING

We suggest you only use the following herbs under the supervision of a professional herbalist.

Barberry

Bugleweed: can reduce milk production

Cats Claw

Cayenne

Dan Shen

Elecampane

False Unicorn Root

Feverfew

Garlic: usually fine, though can cause loose stools in some infants

Ginger

Ginseng (but *Siberian Ginseng* is safe)

Golden Seal

Guaicum

Holy Thistle

Horehound (*Black* and *White*)

Horsetail

Juniper

Liquorice

Meadowsweet: high in salicylates which can cause allergy

Myrrh

Nutmeg

Oregon Mountain Grape

Passionflower

Peony

Peppermint: can reduce milk production

Periwinkle (and all *Vinca* species)

Poplar: high in salicylates which can cause allergy

Saw Palmetto

Schisandra

Shatavari

St John's Wort

Tansy

Tea-Tree oil: if used on nipple wash off before feeding

Thyme

Uva Ursi

Valerian

Vinca (all species)

Vervain

Wild Indigo

Wild Yam

Willow: high in salicylates which can cause allergy

Yarrow

Herbs which contain essential oils

Essential oils (if used on nipple wash off before feeding)

Any herbs with hormonal activity

Laxative herbs may cause loose stools in infant

Sedative herbs may cause drowsiness in infant and increase risk of
SIDS

Herbs which contain phyto-oestrogens. Some of these, such as *Alfalfa*,
Fennel and *Red Clover* are safe to take in the short term to increase
breast milk.

Herbs which have a diuretic action. You need to be well hydrated to
breastfeed successfully.

HERBS WHICH SHOULD NOT BE USED WHILE BREASTFEEDING

Aconitum

Aloe species

American Hellebore (Veratrum)

*American Mandrake
(Podophyllum)*

Ammi Visnaga

Andrographis

Belladonna

Bittersweet (and all *Solanum*
species)

Black Cohosh

Bladderwrack

Blue Cohosh

Blue Flag

Bogbean

Boldo

Boneset

Borage

Bracken Fern (Pteridium)

Broom

Bryonia

Buckthorn

Cascara Sagrada

Castor Bean: will reduce milk
flow

Chapparal

Coltsfoot

Comfrey

Conium

Convallaria (Lily of the Valley)

Corydalis ambigua

Cotton Root

Culvers Root

Datura (Johnson Weed)

Digitalis

Embelia ribes

Ephedra (Ma huang)

False Hellebore

Ferula

Fumitory

Gelsemium

Germander

Greater Celandine

Jasmine Flower: will reduce milk
flow

Johnson Weed (Datura)

Kava Kava

Life Root

Lily of the Valley (Convallaria)

Lobelia

Lomatium

Lupinus

Ma huang (Ephedra)

Mistletoe

Nicotiana (Tobacco)

Oleander

Papaver somniferum (Poppy)

Peach Tree

Pennyroyal

Phytolacca (Poke Root)

Pleurisy Root

Podophyllum (American
Mandrake)

Poison Ivy

Poke Root (Phytolacca)

Poppy (Papaver somniferum)

Prickly Ash

Prunus species

Pteridium (Bracken Fern)

Pulsatilla

Rauwolfia

Rhubarb: safe to eat as a food

Sage: will reduce milk flow

Sanguinaria

Sassafras

Senecia

Senna

Solanum (all species)

Sorghum

Squill

Sweet Flag

Thuja

Tobacco (Nicotiana)

Trachymene

Veratrum (American Hellebore)

Wahoo

Wild Carrot

Wild Cherry

Wintergreen

Yellow Dock

Any plant to which you are
allergic

Herbs which are central nervous
system stimulants, e.g. coffee

Safety of diseases and infections during breastfeeding

There are some diseases and infections which can be transmitted through breast milk and others which can't. In some instances, HIV for example, there is controversy, and different studies suggest different outcomes. We've listed here some conditions which may concern you, but this list does *not* replace the advice of a medical practitioner. Remember, too, that breastfeeding confers considerable immune protective support to your baby, and this needs to be a part of any decision you make as to whether you breastfeed or not.

Chickenpox   the virus is transferred through breast milk. The main danger occurs when the onset of the disease is within five days prior to delivery or two days after. Seek medical advice as your baby may need treatment.

Cytomegalovirus   crosses into the milk, but this is often a past infection and the baby may already have antibodies. Get medical advice.

Hepatitis A   you should be able to continue to breastfeed unless you are acutely ill or jaundiced. Get medical advice on treatment for you and your baby.

Hepatitis B   can be transmitted through milk but you may be able to continue to feed after medical treatment for you and your baby.

Hepatitis C transmission through breast milk is possible but not documented. There is a danger of infection from bleeding around the nipples. Get medical advice.

Herpes 1 and 2 have been isolated in breast milk even in the absence of lesions and, although this does not appear to be a common mode of transmission, some cases have been documented. Lesions on the breast or nipple must be covered. Get medical advice and see our book *Healthy Body, Better Birthing* for natural remedies.

HIV the evidence seems to support the idea that HIV is transmitted from mother to child through breast milk. This applies to mothers who become infected while breastfeeding. It is not clear whether the virus is transmitted through breast milk if the mother was infected prior to pregnancy. However, one considerable study from South Africa suggests that breastfeeding helps to protect the baby from the mother's HIV infection. The exact risk is not known and you should seek medical advice.

Insect stings most probably do not penetrate into breast milk. Even if they did, the toxins would probably be destroyed by the infant's stomach acid. However if you are severely affected or your baby seems to be unwell, seek medical advice.

Lyme disease the disease is transmitted via breast milk and can cause infection in the infant. Seek medical advice.

The glycaemic index

There are two types of carbohydrates: risk-reducing (low glycaemic) and risk-promoting (high glycaemic). Which category a food falls into depends on the amount of carbohydrate present in the food and the amount of fibre it contains. Foods that are low in carbohydrate and high in fibre or water are risk-reducing or low glycaemic, and it is those foods you should select whenever possible. The moderate risk foods may be eaten, but in smaller amounts.

LOW GLYCAEMIC FOODS: EAT MOST

apples
apricots
asparagus
berries
bok choy
broccoli
brussel sprouts
cabbage
capsicum
cauliflower

chickpeas
cucumbers
eggplants
grapes
kidney beans
lentils
lettuce
melons (but not watermelon, which is high in sugar)
mushrooms

onions

oranges

peaches

pineapples

spinach

strawberries

tomatoes

HIGH GLYCAEMIC FOODS: EAT IN MODERATION

baked beans

bananas

biscuits

bread

carrots

corn

dates

figs

fruit juices

grains*

mangoes

muffins

papaya

pasta

peas

potatoes

relishes

rice

squash

sweet potatoes

tacos

tortillas

watermelon

* With the exception of Basmati rice, all refined (white) grains have a higher rating than the wholegrain variety.

How to use natural remedies

HERBAL MEDICINE

If you visit a herbalist, your herbal medicine is likely to be given as a fluid extract or tincture (liquid preparations), tablets or capsules, and the practitioner will set the appropriate dosage.

If you are self-medicating (following the advice given here) it's easier and safer to use herbal infusions or herbal teas, though to be effective herbs need to be infused (or the teabag left in the water) for at least 15 minutes.

How to make and use an infusion

1. For every 30 grams (2 tablespoons) of herb, pour on 600 mL of boiling water.
2. Let it steep (infuse) for at least 15 minutes to get the full benefit of the active ingredients of the herb.
3. Strain the mixture and retain the liquid.
4. Drink a cupful three times daily.
5. Make a fresh brew every day and use it within 24 hours or refrigerate.

While infusions are not as strongly active in most cases as the preparations you will receive from a herbalist, they can still be very effective, and in some cases are the preferred forms. Although you will find you can treat mild conditions easily yourself, any severe or continuing problem requires professional diagnosis and treatment.

You will also find many herbal medicines in tablet or capsule form in health food shops, and these should have clear directions (and cautions for breastfeeding) on the label. The staff in these shops may also be able to help you, but we recommend strongly that you check all herbal preparations, whatever form they may take, against the list of contraindicated herbs in Appendix 2.

Information on herbal medicine is very comprehensive and thorough these days. Not only is there a substantial and growing body of scientific research into the constituents and effects of herbs, but there is also the advantage of experience gathered over many centuries of traditional use.

ACUPUNCTURE AND ACUPRESSURE

The uses of acupuncture are many and varied, and in the hands of a skilled practitioner acupuncture can be an excellent way to treat almost any condition.

For self-help, acupressure is the easiest approach, and in the text we recommend specific points that can be used to treat many of the conditions of breastfeeding. You may wish to investigate one of the hand-held acupressure machines that are on the market which deliver an electrical impulse. Some of these even have an indicator which lights up as you hit the right spot.

How to stimulate an acupressure point

First, find the point as accurately as you can, then apply pressure in the appropriate way. Choose from the three methods below, unless specific instructions are given.

Calming
Cover the point with the palm of the hand or gently stroke it for about two minutes. This method should be used when there is overactivity involved in the condition, such as stress.

Tonifying
Apply stationary or clockwise pressure for two minutes. This pressure

can be slowly increased as your tolerance to discomfort increases. (Points relating to an organ or condition in need of treatment may be tender.) Pressing too hard straight away can cause you to tense. Gradually increased pressure can be better tolerated and therefore more easily built up to effective levels. This method should be used for sluggish or depressed conditions.

Dispersing

Apply moving pressure such as a circular anticlockwise motion or a pumping action in and out on the point. The pressure can be begun fairly deep and then brought up to the surface. Take care to keep the area relaxed, and increase the pressure during successive treatments as you learn to tolerate it. This method should be used if there is congestion.

REFLEXOLOGY

Reflexology is similar to acupressure, as it involves pressure to trigger points. In reflexology these points, or zones, are located on the feet or hands, and can be stimulated, or calmed, in the same way as described above for acupressure.

HOMOEOPATHY

Homoeopathy works by using minute amounts of herbal or mineral substances to trigger a response in the body, and although the small amounts are not in themselves toxic, the responses they trigger can sometimes be quite powerful (as can the healing effects!).

Homoeopathic remedies are particularly appropriate during breast-feeding, and we have recommended their use several times in this book. However, apart from the specific instances that we have noted, you should always consult a qualified homoeopath and not attempt to choose remedies for yourself. Where we have given alternatives, the choice of remedy can be made either by consulting a practitioner or referring to a specific homoeopathic text.

Checklist: how to reduce the toxins in breast milk

- Ventilate your house well
- Don't lose a lot of weight (as fat breaks down, toxins are released)
- Take in sufficient kilojoules
- Eat organically-grown or fed food
- Don't store food in tins or plastic containers
- Eat nutritious food
- Don't microwave your food
- Drink fresh vegetable juices
- Wash fruit and vegetables in vinegar and water (1 tablespoon to 500 mL). Do not soak as this leaches nutrients
- Avoid eating large fish, or those from river and coastal waters
- Avoid eating bottom-dwelling fish and crustaceans
- Trim all fat from foods
- Use a water purifier for all your drinking water and cooking
- Avoid tetra packs
- Don't use aluminium cookware
- Don't cook or keep high-acid foods in metal containers
- Avoid caffeine
- Avoid cigarettes and passive smoking

- Avoid alcohol
- Don't exercise too strenuously
- Avoid unnecessary medications
- Use antioxidants
- Supplement wisely
- Use non-toxic cleaning materials
- Close windows in heavy traffic
- Grow plants in your home
- Wipe your feet or remove your shoes on entering your house
- Avoid solvents, paints and glues
- Don't dry-clean clothes (or at least air them well before wearing)
- Replace foam-based furniture
- Replace synthetic or treated carpet
- Avoid pesticide and fertiliser use
- Use natural toiletries
- Don't use anti-perspirant sprays
- Avoid antacids
- Check exposure to chemicals or toxins at work. Use all protective measures possible.
- Put net curtains over windows facing busy roads
- Avoid oral contraceptives and IUDs containing copper
- Keep electrical gadgets out of the bedroom
- Switch to a laptop or limit computer monitor exposure
- Try not to fly too often
- Avoid X-rays
- Don't stand by the photocopier for extended periods
- Limit use of mobile phones

And, above all, enjoy your breastfeeding relationship. It's one of the golden periods in your life!

Recommended reading

Throughout this book we have referred to numerous studies and research. Although there is not room here to cite specific references, you will find all the relevant information in the books and journals recommended below. Specific enquiries can be directed to the authors

c/- Newleaf
Gill & Macmillan Publishers
Hume Avenue
Park West
Dublin 12
Ireland

For a comprehensive catalogue of titles on breastfeeding and all related topics contact:

CAPERS, PO Box 412, Red Hill, QLD 4059; Ph: (61-7) 3369 9200,
Fax: (61-7) 3369 9299, Email: jan@capersbookstore.com.au

For a comprehensive catalogue of all titles on nutritional and environmental medicine contact:

Australian College of Nutritional & Environmental Medicine,
13 Hilton St, Beaumaris, VIC 3193; Ph: (61-3) 9589-6088,
Fax: (61-3) 9589 5158

Other suggested titles include:

Breastfeeding

Balaskas, Janet & Yehudi, Gordon. *The Encyclopaedia of Pregnancy and Birth*. Little, Brown and Co Ltd, UK, 1992.

Cox, Sue. *Breastfeeding: I Can Do That*. TasLaC, Australia, 1997.

Kitzinger, Sheila. *Breastfeeding*. Dorling Kindersley, UK, 1989.

La Leche International. *The Womanly Art of Breastfeeding*. Universal-Tandem, USA, 1971.

Moody, J., Britten, J. & Higg, K. *Breastfeeding Your Baby*. Fisher Books, National Childbirth Trust, UK, 1997.

O'Brien, P. *Discovering Childbirth & the Joy of Breastfeeding*. Angus & Robertson, Australia, 1979.

Renfrew, Fisher & Arms. *Bestfeeding*. Celestial Arts, USA, 1990.

Stewart, Maryon. *Healthy Parents, Healthy Baby*. Headline, UK, 1995.

Nutrition

Bland, J. *Nutraerobics*. Harper & Row, USA, 1983.

Baker, D.J.P. *Mothers, Babies and Health in Later Life*. Churchill Livingstone, UK, 1998.

Brostoff, J. & Gamlin, L. *The Complete Guide to Food Allergy & Intolerance*. Bloomsbury, UK, 1994.

Cheraskin, E., Ringsdorf, W. M. & Clark, J.W. *Diet & Disease*. Keats Publishing, Connecticut, USA, 1968.

Davies, S. & Stewart, A. *Nutritional Medicine*. Pan Books, London, UK, 1987.

Davis, A. *Let's Have Healthy Children*. Allen & Unwin, London, UK, 1968.

Hoffer, A. & Walker, M. *Orthomolecular Nutrition*. Keats Publishing, Connecticut, USA, 1978.

Jennings, I.W. *Vitamins in Endocrine Metabolism*. Heinemann, London, UK, 1970.

Osiecki, Henry. *Nutrients in Profile*. Bioconcepts Publishing, QLD, 1995.

Pfeiffer, C. *Mental and Elemental Nutrients*. Keats Publishing, USA, 1975.

Pfeiffer, C. *Zinc and the Other Micronutrients*. Pivot Original Health, Keats Publishing, USA, 1978.

Price, W.A. *Nutrition and Physical Degeneration*. Price Pottenger Nutrition Foundation, California, USA, 1945.

Sears, Barry. *Enter The Zone*. Harper Collins, NY, 1995.

Watts, David L. *Trace Elements and Other Essential Nutrients*. Writers B-L-O-C-K, USA, 1995.

Werbach, M. *Nutritional Influences on Illness*. Third Line Press, California, USA, 1988.

Williams, R. *Nutrition Against Disease*. Bantam Books, USA, 1971.

Foresight publications (available from the Foresight Association—see Contacts & Resources):

> *The Adverse Effects of Food Additives on Health*
> *The Adverse Effects of Zinc Deficiency*

Recipe books

Alexander, Stephanie. *The Cook's Companion*. Penguin, Australia, 1997.

Brighthope, I. et al. *A Recipe for Health: Nutrient Dense Recipes*. McCullogh, Carlton, VIC, 1989.

Grant, Airdre. *The Good Little Cookbook*. MacPlatypus Productions, Australia, 1998.

Hay, D. & Bacon, Q. *At My Table—Fresh & Simple*. Barbara Beckett, Australia, 1995.

Katzen, M. *Moosewood Cookbook*. Simon & Schuster, Australia, 1997.

Katzen, M. *Moosewood Restaurant Cooks at Home*. Simon & Schuster, Australia, 1994.

Katzen, M. *Moosewood Restaurant Kitchen Garden*. Simon & Schuster, Australia, 1992.

Katzen, M. *New Recipes from Moosewood Restaurant*. Simon & Schuster, Australia, 1997.

Katzen, M. *Sundays at Moosewood Restaurant*. Simon & Schuster, Australia, 1991.

Kilham, Chris. *The Whole Food Bible*. Inner Traditions, UK, 1997.

Milan, Lindley. *Plates*. New Holland, Australia, 1995.

Ombauer, Irma S. *The Joy of Cooking*. Simon & Schuster, Australia, 1998.

Solomon, Charmaine. *The Complete Asian Cookbook*. Lansdowne Publishing, Australia, 1992.

Solomon, Charmaine. *The Complete Vegetarian Cookbook*. Harper Collins, Australia, 1990.

Squirrels Cookbook. Squirrels Publishing, Brisbane, QLD, 1994.

Herbal and Natural Medicine

Airola, P. *Hypoglycemia: A Better Approach*. Health Plus Publishers, Arizona, USA, 1977.

Alexander, P. *It Could Be Allergy and It Can Be Cured*. Ethicare, Sydney, NSW, 1988.

Bone, K. *Clinical Applications of Ayurvedic and Chinese Herbs*. Phytotherapy Press, QLD, 1996.

Bone, K., Burgess, N. & McLeod, D. *How to Prescribe Herbal Medicines*. Mediherb, QLD, 1990.

Buist, R. *Food Chemical Sensitivity*. Harper & Row, Australia, 1986.

Buist, R. *Food Intolerance*. Angus & Robertson (HarperCollins), Sydney, NSW, 1990.

Chapman, E. *The 12 Tissue Salts*. Thorsons, UK, 1960.

De Ruyter, P. *Coping with Candida*. Allen & Unwin, Sydney, NSW, 1989.

Grieve, M. *A Modern Herbal*. Penguin, UK, 1977.

Gustalson, H. & O'Shea, M. *The Candida Directory and Cookbook*. Celestial Arts, Berkely, California, USA, 1994.

Hyne Jones, T.W. *Dictionary of the Bach Flower Remedies*. C.W. Daniel Co. Ltd, UK, 1976.

Ingham, E.D. *Stories the Feet Have Told Through Reflexology*. Ingham Publishing Inc., USA, 1951.

Kaminski, P. & Katz, R. *The Flower Essence Repertory*. The Flower Essence Society, California, USA, 1994.

Mills, S. *Dictionary of Modern Herbalism*. Thorsons, UK, 1985.

Mills, S. *The Essential Book of Herbal Medicine*. Arkana, UK, 1991.

Mills, S. & Bone K. *Principles and Practice of Phytotherapy*. Churchill Livingstone, UK, 2000.

Oghashi, W. *Do-It-Yourself Shiatsu*. Unwin, UK, 1979.

Segal, M. *Reflexology*. Wilshire Book Company, California, USA, 1976.

Sichel, G. & M. *Relief from Candida, Allergies and Ill Health*. Sally Milner Publishing, Sydney, NSW, 1990.

Stuart, M. *Encyclopedia of Herbs and Herbalism*. Orbis, London, UK, 1979.

Turner, R. & Simonsen, E. *Candida Can Be Beaten*. Oidium Books, Geelong, VIC, 1985.

Werbach, M.R. *Botanical Influences on Illness*. Third Line Press, California, USA, 1994.

Natural Remedies for Women and Children

Airola, P. *Everywoman's Book*. Health Plus Publishers, Arizona, USA, 1979.

Boston Women's Health Collective. *The New Our Bodies, Ourselves*. Penguin, UK, 1989.

Bove, Mary. *An Encyclopaedia of Natural Healing for Children and Infants*. Keats Publishing, Connecticut, USA, 1996.

Brightlight, Elyane. *Natural Childcare*. Brolga Publishing P/L, Ringwood, VIC, 1999.

Cabot, S. *Women's Health*. Pan Books, Sydney, NSW, 1987.

Curtis, S. & Fraser, R. *Natural Healing for Women*. Pandora, UK, 1991.

Harding, M.E. *Women's Mysteries, Ancient & Modern*. Harper & Row, NY, 1976.

Howard, J. *Bach Flower Remedies for Women*. C.W. Daniel, UK, 1992.

Llewellyn-Jones, D. *Everywoman*. Faber & Faber, London, UK, 1971.

Maury, Dr E.A. *Homoeopathic Treatment of Children's Ailments*. Thorsons, UK, 1978.

McQuade-Crawford, Amanda. *Herbal Remedies for Women*. Prima Publishing, USA, 1997.

Melville, A. *Natural Hormone Health*. Thorsons, UK, 1970.

The New Women's Health Handbook. Virago, UK, 1978.

Northrup, Dr Christiane. *Women's Bodies, Women's Wisdom*. Judy Platkus Ltd, London, UK, 1998.

Parvati, J. Hygeia: *A Women's Herbal*. Freestone, USA, 1979.

Reid, Elsa & Enzer, Suzanne. *Maternity Reflexology*. Born to be Free & Soul to Sole Reflexology, Sydney, NSW, 1997.

Reuben, C. & Priestly, J. *Essential Supplements for Women*. Thorsons, UK, 1991.

Rogers, Carol. *The Women's Guide to Herbal Medicine*. Hamish Hamilton, London, UK, 1995.

Romm, Aviva Jill. *Natural Healing for Babies and Children*. The Crossing Press, California, USA, 1996.

Rose, Dr B. & Scott-Moncrieff, Dr C. *Homoeopathy for Women*. Harper Collins, UK, 1998.

Somer, Elizabeth. *Nutrition for Women—The Complete Guide*. Henry Holt, NY, 1993.

Speight, P. *Homoeopathic Remedies for Women's Ailments*. Health Science Press, UK, 1985.

Tisserand, M. *Aromatherapy for Women*. Thorsons, UK, 1985.

Trickey, Ruth. *Women, Hormones and the Menstrual Cycle*. Allen & Unwin, Sydney, NSW, 1998.

Trickey, Ruth & Cooke, Kaz. *Women's Trouble*. Allen & Unwin, Australia, 1998.

Weed, Sussan. *Wise Woman Herbal for the Childbearing Year*. Ash Tree Publishing, NY, 1986.

Natural Fertility Management

Billings, E. & Westmore, A. *The Billings Method*. Anne O'Donovan, Melbourne, VIC, 1980.

Naish, F. *The Lunar Cycle*. Nature & Health Books, Australia and New Zealand; Prism Press, UK, 1989.

Naish, F. *Natural Fertility*. Sally Milner Publishing, Sydney, NSW, 1991.

Ostrander, S. & Shroeder, L. *Astrological Birth Control*. Prentice-Hall, New Jersey, USA, 1972.

Lifestyle/Environmental Factors

Archer, John. *The Water You Drink: How Safe Is It?* Purewater Press, Australia, 1996.

Ashton, J. & Laura, R. *The Perils of Progress: The Health and Environment Hazards of Modern Technology and What You Can Do About Them*. University of New South Wales Press, Sydney, NSW, 1998.

Colborn, Theo, Myers, John Peterson & Dumanoski, Dianne. *Our Stolen Future*. Dutton, USA, & Little Brown & Co., UK, 1996.

Elkington, J. & Haile, J. *The Green Consumer Guide*. Penguin Books, Australia, 1989.

Hodges, J. *Harvesting the Suburbs*. Nature & Health Books, Australia, 1985.

Ott, J. *Health and Light*. Pocket Books, Simon & Schuster, New York, USA, 1976.

Powerwatch. *Living with Electricity*. Powerwatch, 2 Tower Road, Sutton, Ely, CB62QA Cambridgeshire, UK.

Salminen, S. et al. *Safeguards (Home Chemicals Guide)*. McPhee Gribble (Penguin), Melbourne, VIC, 1991.

Smith, R. & Total Environment Centre. *Chemical Risks and the Unborn: A Parents Guide*. Total Environment Centre, Sydney, 1991.

Foresight publications (available from the Foresight Association—see Contacts & Resources):

The Adverse Effects of Alcohol on Reproduction
The Adverse Effects of Tobacco Smoking on Reproduction
The Adverse Effects of Lead
The Adverse Effects of Agrochemicals on Reproduction and Health

Health Issues from an Holistic Perspective

The following is a list of journals and newsletters which report on studies and research findings regarding health issues from an holistic perspective. Many of the studies we have mentioned have been reported in these journals.

Proof!, What Doctors Don't Tell You & Natural Parent
    WDDTY, Satellite House, 2 Salisbury Road, London SW19 4EZ, UK;
    Ph: (44-2) 8944 9555, Fax: (44-2) 8944 9888,
    Email: wddty@zoo.co.uk, Website: www.wddty.co.uk
International Journal of Alternative & Complementary Medicine
    Green Library, 9 Rickett Street, Fulham, London, UK; Ph: (44-171)
    385 0012, Fax: (44-171) 385 4566
Clinical Pearls News
    I.T. Services, 3301 Alta Arden #2, Sacramento, CA 95825, USA;
    Ph: (1-916) 483 1085, Fax: (1-916) 483 1431
Environment & Health News
    The Environment Health Trust, PO Box 1954 , Glastonbury, Somerset
    BA6 9FE, UK; Ph: (44-176) 762 7038
Australian Journal of Medical Herbalism
    National Herbalists' Association of Australia, PO Box 403, Morisset,
    NSW 2264; Ph: (61-2) 4973 4107, Fax: (61-2) 4973 4857,
    Email: ajmh@nhaa.org.au, Website: www.nhaa.org.au
Journal of the Australian Traditional-Medicine Society
    ATMS, PO Box 1027, Meadowbank, NSW 2114; Ph: (61-2) 9809
    6800, Fax: (61-2) 9809 7570, Email: enquiries@atms.com.au,
    Website: www.atms.com.au
The Natural Therapist
    Australian Natural Therapists' Association, PO Box 856, Caloundra,
    QLD 4551; Ph: (61-7) 5491 9850, Fax: (61-7) 5491 5679,
    Email: ANTA1955@bigpond.com
Health & Wellness Report
    Tapestry Communications, Spectrum Marketing Services, PO Box
    264, Toorak ,VIC 3142; Ph: (61-3) 8247 7938

Life Spirit & Natural Health Review
    PO Box 312, Fortitude Valley, QLD 4006; Ph: (61-7) 3854 1286,
    Fax: (61-7) 3252 4579, Email: nhr@nhr.com.au
Herbalgram
    American Botanical Council & Herb Research Foundation, PO Box
    201660, Austin, Texas 78720, USA; Ph: (1-512) 331 8868
Alternative Medicine Review
    Thorne Research Inc., 25820 Highway 2 West, Sandpoint,
    ID 83864, USA; Ph: (1-208) 263 1337, Fax: (1-208) 265 2488,
    Email: kelly@thorne.com
Alternative Medicine Digest
    Future Medicine Publishing Inc. Editorial Office, 21½ Main Street,
    Tiburon, California 94920, USA; Ph: (1-415) 789 8700
Australian Health & Healing
    Australian Health Newsletters, PO Box 427, Paddington, NSW 2021
Journal of Health Sciences
    PO Box 6200, South Penrith, NSW 2750
*Alternative and Complementary Therapies, The Journal of Alternative
and Complementary Medicine, Journal of Womens' Health and
Gender-Based Medicine, & Journal of Medicinal Food*
    Mary Ann Liebert Inc, 2 Madison Avenue, Larchmont, NY 10538,
    USA; Ph: (1-914) 834 3100, Fax: (1-914) 834 1388, Website:
    www.liebertpub.com
Journal of Nutritional & Environmental Medicine
    Carfax Publishing Ltd, Rankine Road, Basingstoke, Hants RG24
    8PR, UK
*The Journal of the Australasian College of Nutritional & Environmental
Medicine*
    ACNEM, 13 Hilton Street, Beaumaris, VIC 3193; Ph: (61-3) 9589
    6088, Fax: (61-3) 9589 5158
International Clinical Nutrition Review
    Integrated Therapies, PO Box 370, Manly NSW, 2095
Soma Newsletter
    PO Box 7180, Bondi Beach, NSW 2026; Ph:(61-2) 9789 4805,
    Fax: (61-2) 9922 5747
Birthings
    Homebirth Access Sydney, PO Box 66, Broadway, NSW 2007

Birth Issues

Capers, PO Box 412, Red Hill, QLD 4059; Ph: (61-7) 3369 9200, Fax: (61-7) 3369 9299

Breastfeeding Review

Australian Breastfeeding Association, PO Box 4000, Glen Iris, VIC 3146; Ph: (61-3) 9885 0855

Journal of Human Lactation

Imprint Publications, Inc. 230 East Ohio St, Suite 300, Chicago, IL 60611, USA; Ph: (1-312) 337 9268, Fax: (1-312) 337 9622

Contacts and resources

Francesca and Jan offer the following services that can augment and update the information in this book.

BOOKS IN THIS SERIES

* *Healthy Parents, Better Babies* by Francesca Naish and Janette Roberts, Newleaf
* *Healthy Lifestyle, Better Pregnancy* by Francesca Naish and Janette Roberts, Newleaf
* *Healthy Body, Better Birthing* by Francesca Naish and Janette Roberts, Newleaf

These books are available through all good book stores or through the Internet.

OTHER BOOKS

* *Natural Fertility: The Complete Guide to Avoiding or Achieving Conception* by Francesca Naish, Sally Milner Publishing, $AUS30.00
* *The Lunar Cycle* by Francesca Naish, Nature & Health Books, $AUS12.00

For either of the above books, send credit card details (Visa/Mastercard/Bankcard) to:

Natural Fertility Management
    PO Box 786 Castlemaine
    VIC 3450
    Australia

Ph: 61 3 5472 4922, Fax: 61 3 5470 5766

Or order through: www.fertility.com.au

Email: enquiries@fertility.com.au

There is a charge for postage and packing of $AUS25.00 for 1-4 books.

NATURAL FERTILITY MANAGEMENT

Francesca is the director of Natural Fertility Management which offers the following services through the NFM website: www.fertility.com.au

Or you can write to:

The International Coordinator

Natural Fertility Management

PO Box 786

Castlemaine VIC 3450

Australia

Ph: 61 3 5472 4922, Fax: 61 3 5470 5766

for an NFM contact near you, or details of our postal services.

Natural Fertility Management offers programs for:

- Contraception
- Conscious conception
- Overcoming fertility problems

These programs can be easily followed through our correspondence service, which gives detailed instruction in the use of mucus, temperature and lunar methods, as well as extensive naturopathic and herbal advice for reproductive health. If you wish for more individual recommendations, there is an option to order personal advice, as well as the kit. The kit includes:

- A copy of the book *Natural Fertility – A complete guide to avoiding or achieving conception* (or rebate on proof of purchase).
- An audio cassette with:
  1. Instructions for contraception or conception and use of lunar cycle charts, and
  2. Relaxation techniques, visualisations, and suggestions to assist the synchronization of cycles, increase confidence and motivation, promote reproductive health and general well-being, and deal with stress. In the conception kit there are also suggestions for a healthy conception, pregnancy and birth.
- Blank sympto-thermal charts for recording mucus and temperature and other observations for each menstrual cycle.

- Individual computer-calculated lunar charts showing the potentially fertile times on your personal bio-rhythmic fertility cycle for the next ten years.
- Current year Moon Calendar, showing moon phase present on each day of the year.
- Time zone calculator, to adjust times given on your personal lunar chart for different time zones.
- Attractively bound printed notes for conception or contraception, taking you through the first few months, cycle by cycle.

Options
- For postal or internet clients – detailed written personal advice, including appropriate naturopathic remedies.
- For conscious conception clients – sex selection calculations and advice.
- For clients overcoming fertility problems – male lunar chart, male relaxation and suggestion tape.

Please send for order forms, current fees or addresses of Natural Fertility Management accredited counsellors to the International Coordinator, at the address above, or through the website.

Natural Fertility Management Counsellor Training
Seminars are conducted by Francesca Naish to train health professionals in Natural Fertility Management techniques and the 'Better Babies' program of preconception health care. All accredited counsellors have access to Natural Fertility Management kits for their clients. For details and dates of trainings, contact the International Coordinator, as above.

Natural Fertility Management Nutritional Supplements
NFM has developed a range of practitioner supplements which offer a comprehensive approach to preconception nutritional and detoxification health care. These are available from Nutrition Care, who manufacture the supplements, and can be contacted at:
Nutrition Care Pty Ltd
    25-27 Keysborough Ave
    Keysborough, VIC 3173
    Australia
    Ph: 61 3 9769 0811, Fax: 61 3 9769 0822,
    email: webmaster@nutritioncare.com.au

FORESIGHT ASSOCIATION

Jan is the Australian representative of Foresight, The UK Association for the Promotion of Preconceptual Care. Members receive regular newsletters with updated research results. Fully referenced booklets are available, detailing the adverse effects on reproduction of the following: alcohol, tobacco, zinc deficiency, manganese deficiency, food additives, genito-urinary infections, lead and agrochemicals. The Foresight video 'Preparing for the Healthier Baby' (running time 85 minutes) is suitable for viewing by preconception couples. Information about Foresight practitioners and hair analysis (for toxic metals) is also available. Contact: Foresight (Registered Charity No: 279160)

Mrs. Peter Barnes
28 The Paddock, Godalming, Surrey GU7 1XD
Ph: (01483) 427839
Hours 9.30am-6.00pm
Website: www.foresight-preconception.org.uk

SPA CHAKRA

Jan has developed the Chakra Baby Programs exclusively for Spa Chakra, Australia's premier day spa, with locations in Sydney, Melbourne and Hayman Island. The Chakra Baby program combines a highly interactive range of topics for mother, father and baby, with your choice of one of the Spa's unique mother-baby treatments.

Website: www.chakra.net
email: spachakra@chakra.net

OTHER CONTACTS AND RESOURCES

The following list has been compiled to support the information in Jan and Francesca's books. Further details of other associations, health centres and support groups can be found at

http://www.foresight-preconception.org.uk
http://www.babyonline.com

Action Against Allergy, 24–26 High Street, Hampton Hill, Middlesex TW12 1PD
Action on Smoking and Health (ASHO), 10 Gloucester Place, London W1, Ph: 020 7935 3519

Active Birth Centre, 25 Bickerton Road, London N19 5JT

Active Birth Movement, 52 Dartmouth Park Road, London NW5 1SL

Aqua (Laundry) Washing Balls FREEPHONE 0800 026 0220

Aqualink, 5 Albion Parade, Albion Road, Stoke Newington, London N16 9LD, Ph: 020 7275 9099 (water filters and water deliveries)

Association for Breastfeeding Mothers, Sydenham Green Health Centre, 26 Holmshaw Close, Sydenham, London SE26 4TH

The Association for Holistic Biodynamic Massage Therapy, 20 Oak Drive, Larksfield, Aylesford, Kent ME20 6NU, Ph: 0173 287 5605

The Association for the Improvement of Maternity Services (AIMS), 40 Kingswood Avenue, London NW6 6LS, Ph: 0181 960 5585

Association of Natural Medicine, 19a Collingwood Road, Witham, Essex CM8 2DY, Ph: 0137 650 2762

Association of Radical Midwives (ARM), 62 Greetby Hill, Ormskirk, Lancashire L39 2DT, Ph / Fax: 01695 572776
email: arm@radmid. demon.co.uk

Association of Reflexologists, 27 Old Gloucester Street, London WC1N 3XX, Ph: 0870 567 3320

Biocare, Lakeside, 180 Lifford Lane, Kings Norton, Birmingham B30 3NT, Ph: 0121 433 3727, email: 100574,1017@compuserve.com (nutritional supplements)

Biodynamic Agriculture Association (BDAA), The Painswick Inn Project, Gloucester Street, Stroud, Gloucestershire GL5 IQ6, Ph: 0145 375 9501

British Homoeopathic Association, 27a Devonshire Street, London W1N 1RJ

British Institute for Allergy and Environmental Therapy, Llangwyryfon, Aberystwyth, Dyfed SY23 4EY, Ph: 0197 424 1376

British Osteopathic Association, 8–10 Bolston Place, Marylebone, London NW1 6QH, Ph: 020 7262 5250/1128

British Psychological Society, St Andrews House, 48 Princess Road East, Leicester LE1 7DR, Ph: 0116 254 9568, email: enquiry@bps.org.uk

British Society for Allergy and Environmental Medicine Foundation, PO Box 28, Totton, Southampton

British Society for Nutritional Medicine, PO Box 3AP, London W1A 3AP

Cantassium Company, Green Farm, Larkhall Grove Labs, 225 Putney Bridge Road, London SW15 2PY (nutritional supplements)

Centre for Alternative Technology (CAT), Machynlleth, Powys SY20 9AZ, Ph: 0165 470 2400, email: www.cat.org.uk

Central Register of Advanced Hypnotherapists, Box 14526, London N2 2WG, Ph: 020 7354 9938

CHILD, Charter House, 43 St Leonards Road, Bexhill-on-Sea, East Sussex TN40 1JA, Ph: 0142 473 2361 (infertility support group)

Diagnostic (UK), Cultech Ltd, York Chambers, York Street, Swansea SA1 3NJ, FREEONE 0800 731 5655, email: cultech@btinternet.com (diagnostic and allergy tests and practitioner referral)

Ecos Organic Paints, Lakeland Paints, Ph: 0153 973 2866

Exploring Parenthood, 4 Ivory Place, Treadgold Street, London W11 4BP, Ph: 0171 221 9951, Fax: 0171 221 5501

Family Planning Association, 27–35 Mortimer Street, London W1N 7RJ, Ph: 171 636 7866

Fertility Education Trust, National Secretariat, 24 Selly Wick Drive, Selly Park, Birmingham B29 7JH

Fertility UK, Clitherow House, 1 Blythe Mews, Blythe Road, London W14 ONW, Ph: 020 7371 1341, email: jknight@fertilityuk.org (natural family planning)

FPA UK, 27–35 Mortimer Street, London W1N 7RJ, Ph: 020 7636 7866 (natural family planning)

Fresh Water Filter Company, Gem House, 895 High Road, Chadwell Heath, Essex RM6 4HL., email: mail@freshwaterfilter.demon.co.uk

Guild of Complementary Practitioners, Liddell House, 6 Liddell Close, Finchampstead, Berkshire RG40 4NS, Ph: 0118 973 5757, email: info@gcpnet.com

International Academy of Oral Medicine and Toxicology, Tony Newby President, 72 Harley Street, London W1N 1AE, Ph: 020 7580 3168 (holistic dentists)

International Federation of Aromatherapists (IFA), Stamford House, 2/4 Chiswick High Road, London W4 1TH, Ph: 020 8742 2605

ISSUE, 509 Aldridge Road, Great Barr, Birmingham B44 8NA, Ph: 0121 344 4414 (infertility support group)

Iyengar Yoga Institute, 223a Randolph Avenue, London WC2N 4HS, Ph: 020 7836 5220

La Leche League, Spencer Lester, 30 Whimbrel Way, Banbury, Oxon NW1 7YN, e-mail: www.lalecheleague.org

Maternity Alliance, 59–61 Camden High Street, London NW1 7JL

Midwives Information and Resource Centre, 9 Elmdale Road,Clifton, Bristol BS8 1SL
Customer Services Ph: 0800 581009, e-mail: midirs@dial.pipex.com

Natracare Feminine Hygiene, c/- Bodywise (UK) Ltd, Bristol BS32 4DX, Ph: 0145 461 5500, email: info@natracare.com (unbleached and chemical free tampons and pads)

Natural Parent, 4 Wallace Road, London N1 2PG, Ph: 0171 354 4592, email: wddty@zoo.co.uk (magazine for holistic family living)

Neils Yard Remedies, 15 Neals Yard, Covent Garden, London WC2H 9DP, Ph: 020 7379 7222, email: mail@nealsyardremedies.com (dried herbs and tinctures by mail order)

Nelsons Pharmacy, 73 Duke Street, London W1M 6BY, Ph: 020 7629 3118 (Bach flower remedies)

Organic Advisory Service, Elm Farm Research Centre, Hamstead Marshall, Berkshire RG20 0HR, Ph: 0148 365 7658, email: efrc@compuserve.com

Organic Growers Association, Aeron Park, Llangietho, Dyfed

Organic Information, PO Box 1503, Poole, Dorset BH14 8YE, Ph: 01202 715130

Portland Hospital for Women and Children, 205–209 Great Portland Street, London W1N 6AH, Ph: 0171 580 4400, Fax: 0171 631 1170

Society of Homoeopaths, 2 Artizan Road, Northampton NN1 4HU, Ph: 0160 462 1400

Society for the Promotion of Nutritional Therapy, PO Box 47, Heathfield, East Sussex TN21 8ZX, Ph: 0182 587 2921

Support after Termination for Abnormalities (SAFTA), 29 Soho Square, London W1V 6JB

The Ayurvedic Company of Great Britain, 50 Penywern Road, London SW5 9SX, Ph: 020 7370 2255

The BioElectric Shield, Natures Energy, Nine Elms, Swindon SN5 9UG, Ph: 0179 387 8637 (anti-radiation devices)

The British Acupuncture Council, Park House, 206–208 Latimer Road, London W10 6RE, Ph: 020 8964 0222

The British Chiropractic Association, 29 Whitley Street, Reading, Berkshire RG2 OE9, Ph: 0173 475 7557

The British Herbal Medicine Association, Sun House, Church Street, Stroud, Gloucestershire GL5 1JL, Ph: 0145 375 1389

The British Society for Mercury Free Dentistry, 1 Wellbeck House, 62 Wellbeck Street, London W1M 7HB, Ph: 020 7486 3127

The Dr Bach Foundation, Mount Vernon, Sotwell, Wallingford, Oxon OX10 OP2, Ph: 0149 183 4678 (Bach flower remedies)

The European Shiatsu Network, Highbanks, Lockeridge, Marlborough, Wiltshire SN8 4EQ, Ph: 0167 286 1362

The Green People Company, Brighton Road, Hardcross, West Sussex RH17 6BZ, Ph: 0144 440 1444 (mail order tinctures and environmentally safe, personal care products)

The Kinesiology Federation, PO Box 83, Sheffield S7 2YN, Ph: 0114 281 4064

The Moon Calendar Company, PO Box 3081, Bath BA1 5BH, Ph: 0122 586 8850, www.mooncalendar.co.uk (lunar calendar)

The Natural Maid Company, Unit D7, Maws Craft Centre, Jackfield, Ironbridge, Shropshire TF8 7LS, Ph: 0195 288 3288, email: paint@livos.demon.co.uk (non-toxic paints and other products)

The Soil Association, Bristol House, 40–56 Victoria Street, Bristol BS1 6BY, Ph: 0117 929 0661, email: info@soilassociation.org

The Tai Chi Union for Great Britain, 69 Kilpatrick Gardens, Clarkston, Glasgow G76 7RF

Taoist Tai Chi Centre, Bounstead Road, Blackheath, Colchester, Essex CO2 0DE, Ph: 1206 576167

Toxoplasmosis Trust, 61–71 Collier Street, London N1 9BE, Ph: 0171 713 0663

Vaginal Birth After Caesarean (VBAC) Support Group, 8 Wren Way, Farnborough, GU14 8SZ, Ph: 01252 543250

Vitamin Service, Dellrose Cottage, Littlewick Road, Knaphill, Woking, Surrey GU21 2JU, Ph: 01483 488845, Fax: 01483 799574

Wellbeing, The Health Research Charity for Women and Babies, 27 Sussex Place, Regent's Park, London NW1 4SP, Ph: 020 7262 5337

Wholefood, 24 Paddington Street, London W1M 4DR

Index